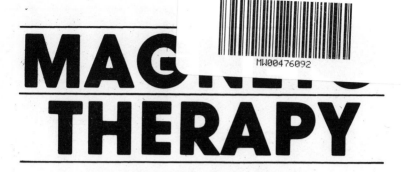
MAGNETO THERAPY

SELF-HELP BOOK

Dr. H. L. BANSAL, *RHMP, MIHL, ARSH,*
Magnetotherapist and Homoeopath,
President: All India Magnetotherapy Association
Director: Indian Institute of Magnetotherapy

&

Dr. R. S. BANSAL

B. Jain Publishers (P) Ltd.
An ISO 9001 : 2000 Certified Company
USA — EUROPE — INDIA

MAGNETO THERAPY – SELF HELP BOOK

First Edition: 1976
Second Edition: 1979
Third Edition (Revised & enlarged): 1987
19th Impression: 2009

NOTE FROM THE PUBLISHERS
Any information given in this book is not intended to be taken as a replacement for medical advice. Any person with a condition requiring medical attention should consult a qualified practitioner or therapist.

Published by Kuldeep Jain for

B. Jain Publishers (P) Ltd.
Available in USA from:
Pjan International, Inc.
800-438-7736

ISBN: 978-81-319-0188-5

Dedicated to

Dr. R.S. Thacker

MY TEACHER
AND
GUIDE IN MAGNETOTHERAPY

PREFACE TO THE THIRD EDITION

This book was originally published in 1976 and contained 176 pages only. It immediately caught attention of the medical profession and the general public, with the result that every year one or more reprints were published. It was also taken note of by the then President and Vice-President of India, in addition to various other celebrities. The response was so good that I reworked on the book, enlarging it to as many as 300 pages in the second edition, published in 1979.

The second edition drew a still wider market, and six years after its publication, we are now publishing a third, revised and enlarged edition. Meanwhile, the book has been published in a Hindi version also, titled 'CHUMBAK CHIKITSA' which has gone into several reprints.

In the present edition, all the acceptable suggestions have been adopted and incorporated. The first sub-head of each chapter has also been printed in this edition.

Electricity has been gaining ground in every sphere including Magnetotherapy. Electromagnets have been introduced in magnet treatment which are relatively more effective in many chronic ailments. A new chapter on 'Electromagnetotherapy' has been added at the end of this edition.

I hope that with the revision and additions mentioned above, the present edition of the book will be fouud more attractive, interesting and useful.

My labour will be amply rewarded if the learned readers patronise this revised and enlarged book and make full use of it by practising Magnetotherapy at their clinics, homes and by extending it to others. I shall, however, welcome experiences and new suggestions for further development of Magnetotherapy.

NEW DELHI   H.L. BANSAL

Foreword

Magnet has proved its indispensability in modern man's technological and industrial ventures. Is it also going to establish itself in the world of modern therapy as a major healing agent ? This treatise by Dr. H. L. Bansal claims it is going to, and he sounds reasonable.

Years back, on a friend's persuation, I took my weeping eczema, deteriorating in spite of best treatment available to me in my position, to Dr. R.S. Thacker, the only magnetotherapist of Delhi known at that time, to whom this book has been appropriately dedicated. I was amazed to get rid of my trouble-some disease in a wonderfully short time. It was this case (quoted in this book on page 153) which inspired Dr. Bansal to go in for Magnetotherapy in a missionary way. This book is the fruit of his devoted labours during the past several years.

In advanced foreign countries, considerable research has been done on the effects of magnetism on the biology of plants, animals and human beings and it has been indisputably established that a number of human ailments could be cured by applying magnets.

One Dr. Maclean, M.D. of New York City, has successfully cured advanced Cancer cases and has made this startling observation : "Cancer cannot exist in a strong magnetic field". The Russians are utilising magnets and magnetised water for curing ailments like mastitis, pains and swellings and even for sufferings caused by the dreaded kindney-stones. The Japanese have manufactured a number of magnetic devices like Magnetic Health Bands, Necklaces, Bed-pads, Belts and even Magnetic chairs for treatment of various diseases.

In India it is seemingly a novel therapy, an amusing one too, but lately a number of physicians, especially Homoeopaths, have adopted it and obtained very encouraging results. Dr. Bansal, basically a homoeopath, has made thorough studies of the results achieved in this field in India as well as in foreign countries. He has experimented extensively and has cured numerous patients of various ailments. And for the benefiit of patients and other physicians, he has produced this book, perhaps first of its kind, written exclusively on the therapeutic use of magnetism providing interesting and useful information on all aspects of the subject, *viz.*, history, principles and practice of magnetotherapy, substantiating it by quoting a large number of treated cases. In addition, he has given guidelines for the treatment of hundred fifty common diseases, which makes the book all the more useful.

This book has made me appreciate the remark of Dr. F.V. Broussais of France, "If magnetism were true, medicine would be an absurdity". And magnetism has been proved to be true as every reader of this book will find for himself.

I congratulate the author for this very useful work done with humanitarian zeal, with the noble purpose of providing an easy cure to the suffering humanity.

K.C. GUPTA
Deputy Secretary (Retd.)
Ministry of Health & Family Planning,
Government of India, New Delhi.

Acknowledgments

I solemnly acknowledge that I owe my indebtedness to Dr. R.S. Thacker, the aged and experienced Magnetotherapist of Kashi Ram Building, Kashi Ram Lane, Dareeba Kalan, Delhi, who attracted me to the field of his magnetic cures and has shared with me his vast knowledge and experiences in the rare technique of healing patients through magnets. He imparted his valuable knowledge of Magnetotherapy to me so that his knowledge and experiences of the past over 25 years might be extended and disseminated for the benefit of the mankind. He is the oldest magnetotherapist in India and has successfully treated thousands of patients, free of charge, during this long period.

My young friend, Dr. M.T. Santwani, Homoeopathician and Magnetotherapist inspired me to take interest in magneto-therapy and his friendly insistence created a deep desire in me to study this subject. My thanks are also due to Dr. A.K. Bhattacharya of Naihati, 24 Parganas, West Bengal, author of the book "Magnet and Magnetic Fields". I also record my thanks to the authors and publishers of other books, journals and articles mentioned in the 'list of references', given at the end.

A word of thanks and appreciation to M/s. B. Jain Publishers, (P) Ltd., New Delhi-110055 who have published this book and have given it wide publicity so that a large number of its readers may make use of healing properties of magnets.

(*x*)

This book has seen many reprints over a period of last ten years and the third revised and enlarged edition is now in your hands.

Clinic   :   18, C. S. C.
               Arjun Nagar, Safdarjung Enclave
               New Delhi—110029
               Phone : 6107417

H.L. BANSAL

Contents

Part I

1

Introduction

Ancient Knowledge about Magnets

Magnetism is well-known in the fields of physics, industry and commerce. It is also known for centuries to have remarkable effects on certain metals as well as on living organisms, but its recognition as having highly beneficial clinical impact on human ailments has been a comparatively recent development and is not yet widely known.

In the past, variety of wonderful properties were attributed to the magnet from time to time. For instance, dignitaries wore magnets on their persons for the purpose of maintaining vigorous health and for arresting ageing of their bodies. Cleopatra (69—30 B.C.), the extraordinarily beautiful daughter of the king of Egypt—Ptolemy Auletes—is said to have worn a magnet on her forehead to maintain her beauty. Magnet was used as an amulet to relieve headaches. The common people believed that the magnet had a divine force. A philosopher-scientist went to the extent of concluding that "a magnet has a soul because it moved iron". Although, apparently, a magnet has no life, yet the intelligence of its poles to recognize friendship or hatred of the poles of another magnet and to attract or repel it accordingly, remains unexplained even today.

Magnet has proved to be highly beneficial in certain diseases. It is known to have the power of drawing pain out of the body, of relieving stiffness of joints and muscles and of removing toothache immediately. It has also the capacity to reduce weight in obesity, to increase height of short-statured boys and girls and to increase intelligence and wisdom, if used for a long time. It also corrects blood pressure and provides immunity against certain diseases of human body by increasing the vitalising secretions of glands.

Magnetotherapy

Keeping in view these and other innumerable positive properties of the magnet and with the objective of deriving the maximum benefit from its qualities, 'Magnetotherapy'—the system of treating patients through the medium of magnets—is discussed in this book.

A Science and an Art

Magnetotherapy is both a science and an art. This is a science as magnetism is similar to, and works on the lines of, electricity ; and its application is an art as it involves the selection of magnets of different strength, to different parts, to relieve different ailments of the body. It is a system of treatment which covers a vast field of therapeutics and can relieve almost all functional defects of the various systems working in the human body.

Magnetotherapy is based on natural laws and principles and is not a magic or miracle. It means carrying out treatment of the sick with application of magnets over the suffering parts of the body, or on the extremities for altering the diseased condition into a state of recovery and complete health.

Magnetotherapy is too vast a subject to be contained in a small book like this, or in any single volume. The subject cannot be mastered by reading books or following written instructions. It can be mastered only by long and arduous practice and experience.

The use of magnets for treatment is not a new system ; there are references about it in the very ancient records of human knowledge. The system has, however, been forgotten and become almost extinct for various reasons. One of the reasons may be the recent faith of people in antibiotics, fancy for the use of costly modern medicines in place of simple and easily available ones, patent tablets or capsules and injections, etc. professed to afford quick relief.

In Advanced Countries

The system of treatment with magnets has, however, been gaining popularity in the advanced countries like USA. USSR,

Japan, and several other countries and a large number of patients, including those suffering from chronic diseases, are being cured by it. It is, therefore, believed that if a large number of people start taking interest in this sytem of treatment, it will spread out again and help to build a happier and healthier world of less sufferings.

Purpose of the Book

The purpose of this book is to invite the attention of the learned men of medical profession and to inform them about the existence of a large scope for further research and exploration in this seemingly new branch of medical science. The general public can also utilise the therapeutic application of the magnetic properties in their sickness and judge for themselves the advantages of magnetism in relieving and curing diseases, even when they are undergoing treatment under any other system or when other systems of medicine have not been able to tackle their diseases successfully or completely.

It is not easily conceivable why magnets with their power to attract and repel are able to bring about cures of human ailments. An effort has been made in this book to explain how the magnets act on the human system to regulate the process of metabolism and how they work through blood and nerves correcting the circulatory system as well as other systems of the body, namely, nervous, respiratory, digestive and urinary, etc.

There are very few books available in India on this system of treatment. So far the available literature does not explain in detail the methodology of application of magnets in different diseases. It merely provides a short description of some cases successfully treated by some physicians in India and abroad. As this system of treatment is yet to be fully developed, there is no uniform procedure for the use of magnets in human sickness According to the available literature, magnets were placed on the affected parts of the body in the past. Consequently. some persons have worn small magnets around their necks like amulets, or on their wrists like wrist-watches, some have worn them around their waists like belly-belts, while some others have worn them over the affected parts of their bodies. Then, the available books do not provide uniform instructions regarding the time limit for the use of the magnets. This has resulted in some patients having applied magnets for several minutes, some for hours, some for days, some for months and some others even continuously for years. All this goes to show that no standard and effective procedure or technique has been developed and universally followed in the treatment through magnets so far.

Suggestion of Standard Method

Although the exact technique of application of magnets depends on the requirement of each individual case, yet some basic knowledge of the principles of application of magnets is necessary to begin with. Hence an attempt has been made in this book to suggest a standard procedure to be followed in carrying out magnetic treatment on scientific lines. The methods and techniques of application of magnets have been arranged in a systematic way which will render them easy and handy to the reader when he wishes to make use of a magnet as a curative device. The persons who wish to adopt magnetotherapy as their hobby or part-time practice for the benefit of the sick, can easily learn the art from this book.

Knowledge and experience are ever-growing and there is always scope for further research and development. Hence, besides the methods of application of magnets suggested in this book, some other ways of using magnets could also be developed No perfection can, therefore, be claimed by anybody in such matters. The methods suggested herein have, however, been found to be quite effective and are, therefore, recommended for adoption.

In fact magnetotherapy has already cured a number of cases of human illness which were considered and declared incurable. A good number of them will be found listed in the experiences of several magnetotherapists given in Chapter 14. In a large number of cases there was no treatment in modern system of medicine except surgical operation but the patients were cured only by external application of magnets—in many cases without any medicine. It is however true that magnetotherapy takes time for treatment of the cases which are purely surgical in nature.

Use of Magnets Upheld by Homoeopathy

The use of magnets has been upheld and recommended by the Founder of Homoeopathy, Dr. Samuel Hahnemann, too. He has also introduced three varieties of magnetic medicines in Homoeopathy. His observations about the magnet and a number of important symptoms, proved and verified by him for the use of the three magnetic medicines, have been included in a separate chapter in this book. No other branch of medical science seems to have made use of magnets for the treatment of human ailments, in a regular way, so far.

There appears to be a close affinity between the principles of magnetotherapy and practice of Acupuncture or Acupressure. The various 'Acupuncture points' could also be considered as 'magnetic points' for application of magnets on the human body. This view has been dealt with in a separate chapter at the end of this book.

Naturopathy

Similarly, naturopathy which utilises the forces of nature including electricity in correcting the various human disorders, shares many common aspects with magnetotherapy. The latter utilises the greatest universal force of magnetism. The detailed discussion on the similarity between the two systems and their approach to disease and health has been given in a separate chapter at the end of this book.

It is hoped that this new approach would stimulate further thinking in the professionals and others, would open up new avenues for scientific research in this field, as the integrated application of the above mentioned allied medical sciences may help to break the disease deadlock in many cases, for the ultimate benefit of the sick humanity.

The arrangement of different chapters in this book has been so made as to take the reader systematically from the early discovery of the magnets to the advanced techniques of cure.

Besides suggesting the general methods of application of magnets, the treatment of about a hundred and fifty common diseases has been specifically advised. This will make the magnetic treatment more easy and practicable. With a view to provide all easily available information, many cases treated successfully in India and abroad have also been included in separate chapters.

It is a known fact that all inventions, fresh devices and new schemes are introduced on the basis of accumulated experiences and experiments of a number of people, sometimes of several generations. Magnetotherapy has also been developed in course of long time and many physicians, researchers and scientists have contributed towards its development. Hence this book contains, besides the author's own observations and experiences, the ideas, statements, views and experiences of many philosophers, physicians and scientists of several countries.

It is requested that the experiences of the persons who use magnets for the relief of suffering humanity, along with any useful suggestions for improvement in this book, may kindly be intimated to the author for doing the needful.   ★

2

Discovery of Magnetism

Reference of Magnets in Vedas

Magnet and its properties were known to the very ancient Aryans. They believed that the magnet, besides having the power of attracting iron, was also endowed with many mystical and curative powers. There is a mention of treatment of some diseases with special sand and stones at several places in the Vedas which are the most ancient religious scriptures of the Hindus.

Relevant Mantras with English Translations

The Atharva Veda, which is the basis of the Ayurvedic system of treatment, deals with the treatment of many diseases. Some of the mantras of the Atharva Veda are quoted below to substantiate the above statement :

Mantras 3 and 4 of Sukta 17 of Kand 1 of Part I of the Atharva Veda pertain to the treatment for stoppage of bleeding with the help of some articles made of sand and are as follows :—

शतस्य धमनीनां सहस्रस्य हिराणाम् ।
अस्थुरिन्मध्यमा इमाः साकमन्ता अरंसत ॥ **3** ॥
परि व: सिकतावती धनूर्वुं हत्यक्रमीत् ।
तिष्ठतेलयता सु॰कम् ॥ **4** ॥

Mantras 2 and 3 of Sukta 35 of Kand 7 of Part III of the Atharva Veda deal with the treatment of women with the help of stones and are as under :—

इमा यास्ते शतं हिराः सहस्रं धमनीरुत ।
तासां ते सर्वीसामहमश्मना बिलमप्यधाम ॥ **2** ॥
परं योनरवरं ते कृणोमि मा त्वा प्रजाभि भून्मोत सूनु: ।
अस्व त्वाप्रजस कृणोम्यइभान ते अपिधान कृणोमि ॥ **3** ॥

The Dictionary meaning of the word Siktavati used in the mantras of Sukta 17 and of the word Ashman used in the mantras of Sukta 35, mentioned above, are as given below :

Sanskrit-Hindi Dictionary

Sikta	= Sand
Siktavati	= Full of sand
Ashman	= Stone, Chamak Patthar (and other things)
Ashmana	= With the stone

Sanskrit-English Dictionary

Sikta	= Sand, gravel, stone
Ashman	= Stone, rock, precious stone, any instrument of stone

It is thus clear that the mantras of Sukta 17 speak of stoppage of bleeding with something full of or made of sand and the mantras of Sukta 35 mention about the treatment of women with some kind of stone.

The English translations of these mantras by Prof. Friedrich Max Muller of Germany, one of the most eminent orientalists, who has translated all the four Vedas and many other Sanskrit and Hindi religious books of India, are given below :

I. Translations of Mantras 3 and 4 of Sukta 17 :

    (3) Of the hundred arteries, and the thousand veins,
          those in the middle here have indeed stood still,
          at the same time, the ends have ceased to flow.

    (4) Around you has passed a great *sandy dike*,
          stand ye still, pray take your case.

II. Translation of Mantras 2 and 3 of Sukta 35 :

    (2) Of these hundred entrails of thine,
          as well as of the thousands canals,
          of all these have I closed
          the openings with a stone.

    (3) The apper part of the womb do I place below,
          there shall come to thee neither off-spring nor birth,
          I render thee sterile and devoid of off-spring,
          a stone do I make into a cover for thee.

The treatment mentioned in the above mantras of the Atharva Veda could not have been carried out by means of ordinary sand or simple stones but only with some special sand and stones having specific healing properties. The common metallic magnets are made from iron-alloys, while ceramic magnets are manufactured from sand, clay, barium and iron oxide. Hence the mention of the words *Siktavati* (meaning sandy) and *Ashma* (meaning chakmak patthar) in the' Vedas and *Lohakant* in other ancient Ayurvedic literature is a sufficient proof that the magnetic stone and its properties were known and used for theapeutic purposes in India since times immemorial.

Discovery of Magnet in Modern Times

In the comparatively modern age, the discovery of magnet is said to have been made several hundred years Before Christ. However, there are different views about the basis of this discovery. One view is that the power of attraction in a piece of rock, called lodestone, was first discovered some 2500 years ago, by a shepherd boy named Magnes. He, while roaming about on Mount Ida, found that his iron-capped staff got struck to the mountain and it became difficult for him to walk away with his iron-stacked sandals. According to that view, the stone was named after the shepherd boy and came to be called 'Magnet'. Another version is that long ago a kind of dark-coloured Iron-ore composed chiefly of iron and oxygen (Fe_3O_4), was found in abundance in Magnesia in Asia Minor. This ore had attractive and directive powers and it derived the name of Magnetite from magnesia where it was first found.

In 800 B.C., the lodestone was known to the Greeks, as a mention of it is found in the works of Aristotle (384—322 B.C.), Plato (429—347 B.C.) and Homar (about 850 B.C.). Plato gives an account of the "Samothracian Rings", which were used in the ceremonies of the Dactyles, a tribe of roving iron workers. These rings were iron-rings magnetised by contact with natural magnets or lodestones.

Later, the Chinese sailors came to know of the directive property of the natural magnet and used it as a compass for finding directions for their ships in early second century (A.D.). They called it Magnetite, leading stone, or briefly, lodestone.

The famous Swiss Alchemist, Physician and Mystic, Phillippus Aureolus Paracelsus (1493—1541 A.D.) made great landmark in the history of magnetism. He explained it as: "That which constitutes a magnet is an attractive force which is beyond our understanding, but which, nevertheless, causes the attraction of iron and other things". He gave the characteristic powers of the magnet, particularly for healing the sick. He observed that the magnet is especially useful in all inflammations, influxes and ulcerations, in the diseases of bowels and uterus, in internal as well as external diseases. The observations recorded by him centuries ago hold good even at present.

Then Dr. William Gilbert of Colchester, England (1540—1603 A.D.), a famous physician of his time, who was also the President of the college of physicians and the court physician to the Queen Elizabeth I, was the first Englishman to make a scientific study of Electricity and Magnetism. He made wide tours and studied the peculiar behaviour of magnetic needle showing different declinations and inclinations and gave out that the earth itself is a huge magnet. He made many experiments to prove his theories. He placed a rod of iron pointing North and South and hammered it so that it became magnetised by earth's influence. In the year 1600 A.D., he wrote an epoch-making book named "De Magnet", which became very popular. While studying this book, Galilei or Galileo (1564—1642), a great mathematician, philosopher and scientist of Itaty, once remarked "I extremely admire and envy the author of "De Magnet". Gilbert also showed that iron ceases to be attracted when red hot and that substances such as paper and cloth do not affect the force of attraction between a magnet and iron. Most of the terms now current in magnetism were used by him, perhaps for the first time.

Then several other scientists made further experiments and gave their experiences to the world. In the middle of the 19th century, Michael Faraday (1791-1867), an English scientist, made very important discoveries and revelations. His first independent achievement was the demonstration of a magnet around a current.

He enriched the science of magnetism in its many branches such as electromagnetism, magnetic lines of force, magnetic rotary polarisation and electromagnetic induction. He kept a careful record of his experimental researches and the last serial number was above sixteen thousand. He is regarded as the founder of Biomagnetics and magnetochemistry. He based his investigations on the earlier researches of the great scientists A.M. Ampere (1775—1836). H.C. Oersted (1777—1851), D.F. Arago (1788—1853) and J.B. Biot (1774—1862). Faraday showed that all matter is magnetic in one sense or the other, that is, the matter is either attracted or repelled by a magnetic field.

First Treatise on Magnetochemistry in India

In India, the first treatise in English dealing with physical principles and the application of Magnetochemistry was produced by Dr. S.S. Bhatnagar and Dr. K.N. Mathur, in the year 1935. They mainly studied oxidation. An excellent summary of the work is given in their book on Magnetochemistry (Macmillan, London—1935).

Dr. S.S. Bhatnagar, M. Sc. (Punjab), D. Sc. (London) made notable contributions to the science of Colloids, surface chemistry, photo-chemistry and magneto-chemistry. He won an award of rupees one lakh which he donated to a University. He was knighted in 1941 and was awarded "Padma Vibhushana" in 1954. He was Director, Scientific and Industrial Research, and Secretary, Ministry of National Resources and Scientific Research, Govt. of India. He expired on the 1st January, 1955.

Further experiments in Biomagnetics and other aspects of magnetotherapy are being made now extensively in many countries like USA, USSR and Japan as well as in India. The foreign countries have already made much advancement in this line. The conclusions arrived at in foreign countries as a result of treatment through magnets are described elsewhere in this book. India has also kept pace with these developments and is making satisfactory progress in this respect, as pointed out in another chapter. Thus the ancient knowledge about the therapeutic uses of the magnet has been revived during the last 200 years and is being developed now with the hope of increasing the utility of magnet as a healer of human sufferings.

Magnet as Known in Different Languages

The original iron-ore, which had attracting power and was natural magnet, was named 'Magnetite'. It was also called 'loadstone' or 'lodestone'. The word loadstone was derived from the word 'load' used in old English, which, among other things, meant course, journey, etc., conveying the idea of direction.

The Greeks called it "Magnetis" or 'Magnesetos' (meaning stone) and the French call it 'Aimant' (meaning magnet and loving).

The magnet is called '*Chumbak*' (kissing stone) in Hindi and '*Maqnatees*' in Urdu and Persian. The Chinese call it '*Chu Shi*' (meaning loving stone).

A big company of Tokyo, Japan, engaged in the manu-facture of various magnetic articles for the treatment of human diseases, has named itself "The Aimante Trading Co. Ltd." after the word 'Aimant'.

Some gemmologists consider a small magnet to be one of the several precious gems which are advised to be worn for various purposes, namely, for maintenance of health, for peace of mind and for general prosperity. Accordingly, they call it a 'Gem' also.

3

Magnetism in the Universe

Earth as a Huge Natural Magnet

Magnetism is the basic principle that dominates and governs the infinite universe and holds various heavenly bodies in a natural bondage. The earth, the sun, the moon and all the other planets in our own galaxy transmit their own magnetic emanations which greatly influence our lives.

The earth is a huge natural magnet and the magnetism of the earth is a very interesting subject. The terrestrial magnetic history is still in the making and full facts about it have not yet been explored and recorded. Hence it is an important field for further research. However, the researches made, results achieved and conclusions reached so far about the magnetism of the earth are summed up below :

The earth exercises its inductive influence on magnetic substances. This fact has been proved through many experiments, as :

(*i*) The anvil of a blacksmith gets magnetised in the North-South direction.

(*ii*) A vertical bar of iron or steel begins to exhibit magnetic properties.

(*iii*) If a bar of iron is laid horizontally in the North-South direction, the end pointing to the North acquires North polarity.

(*iv*) If a magnet is pivoted so as to swing in a vertical plane or in horizontal plane, it comes to rest along particular direction.

All these happen as a result of the inductive influence of the earth and show that the earth behaves as a huge magnet with a magnetic field around it.

In the Northern Hemisphere, the bottom end becomes a North Pole and the top end a South Pole. Reverse is the case in the Southern Hemisphere. In order to have a clear understanding of the state of the earth's magnetism, it is necessary to know the intensity, direction and variation of this great magnetic power over the whole of the surface of the earth and the subject becomes a matter of detailed study. Hence only general and more relevant information about terrestrial magnetism is given here.

Nature of Earth's Magnetism

The earth is transmitting magnetic energy to all living organism—human, animal and plants.

The earth as a natural magnet has two poles, North and South, like those of any ordinary magnet. The North Pole of the earth is located somewhere at the extreme north of North America and the South Pole at the extreme south of South Victoria. The points of the North and the South Poles of the earth do not remain static but undergo slow shifts.

The earth has its magnetic lines of force around it just as an ordinary magnet possesses its magnetic field around it. The magnetic lines of force of the earth extend approximately from the geographical south to the northernly direction. The magnetic cloak or the field of earth is not a thin wrapping round its surface but it forms a thousand mile thick stratum. It has come to light that Sputnik III and other satellites have detected earth's magnetic field extending to a distance of 105600 kilometres (66,000 miles) beyond the surface of the earth. This has been revealed by the presence of the charged particles shot out from the sun and entrapped by the earth's magnetic field.

Whenever we suspend a bar magnet, it points approximately to North and South. It proves that there are two definite regions of the earth which attract the respective opposite poles of the suspended magnet. This happens because the earth is a giganatic magnet with its South Magnetic Pole somewhere near the North Geographical Pole and the North Magnetic Pole near the South Geographical Pole. It is due to the mutual effect of the forces between the Poles of the earth and those of the magnet that the latter tends to set itself parallel to the magnetic axis of the earth. It is, therefore, concluded that the North Geographical Pole and the South Magnetic Pole are near each other, and the North Magnetic Pole is near the South Geographical Pole of the earth. Hence the Geographical Poles of the earth do not coincide with its Magnetic Poles.

For the purpose of marking the poles on a bar magnet, the end of the suspended magnet pointing towards the North Geographical pole of the earth should be marked North Pole and reversely, the end pointing towards the South Geographical pole of the earth as South Pole.

The distribution of magnetic lines of force at various localities of the earth goes to show that the earth behaves very nearly as a uniformly magnetised sphere. Dr. William Gilbert (1540—1603) who carried out certain experiments in the year 1600, gave us the picture of the general character of the earth's magnetic field and concluded that the earth is itself a big natural magnet.

Everything on earth and in the air above is permeated with the earth's magnetic force. Gauss, the illustrious German astronomer, has computed this force and has stated that the attracting force or lifting power of the earth is forty two quintillions and three hundred and ten quadrillions of tons, which, if equally distributed throughout the mass of the earth would make the magnetic intensity of every cubic yard equal to sixty pounds attracting force. Professor Mayor has shown that this magnetic influence is filling space to an unknown distance and is radiating the lines of magnetic force like the rays of the sun.

Sources of Magnetism of Earth

Various theories have been advanced to account for the origin of earth's magnetism. One school of thought is that the earth is a permanently magnetised sphere, having two polarities at the two ends, while the other school of thought is that the annual variations and the magnetic storms of the earth owe their origin to the sun and cause magnetic effect on the earth. Yet another view is that the permanent magnetism of the earth might have its origin in the rotational motions. According to still another view, the magnetic field of the earth may be due to :

(*i*)   a permanent magnet, magnetic masses or electric currents inside the earth,

(*ii*)   a magnetic field, the origin of which is at a considerable distance from the earth,

(*iii*)   electric currents produced due to the ionisation of layers of air surrounding the surface of the earth.

Whatever the source of the magnetism of the earth may be, it has been established in view of what has been stated above, that the earth is a huge natural magnet.

Earth's Magnetic Effect on Human Beings

Human body itself is a magnet. In magnetic parlance, our bodies are considered to have magnetic sides. Considering a human body vertically, the head and the upper half of the body are taken to represent 'North Pole' and their opposites, namely, the feet and the lower half of the body, are taken to represent 'South Pole'. Considering the human body horizontally, the right hand, the right arm and the right side of the body are considered to be 'North Pole' and their opposites, namely, the left hand, the left arm and the left side of the body, are taken to be 'South Pole'. Also the front side of a person consisting of forehead, face, chest and belly is considered North and back side consisting of occiput, back of neck, spine and hips is considered South.

Abiding by natural law and forces, any action or deed done in the natural direction, affords peace and pacification, and causes the least possible discomfort than when done otherwise. Accordingly, if we lie, when going to sleep, in the same posture, in which a hanging bar takes its direction, we can avoid tension, sleeplessness and restlessness. When we lie stretching our North to the North of the earth and our South to the South of the earth, we attain equilibrium. Hence it is wise to lie with the head towards the North and the feet towards the South, while sleeping, specially if one sleeps on the ground. This position brings on better sleep and also improves health. This is because the body in that direction is in accordance with the magnetic direction of the earth and the magnetic currents affect the system favourably.

According to the ancient philosophy, when a person on the death-bed finds it extremely painful and difficult to breath his last, he is made to lie on the earth in the North and South position—the head being towards the North. This brings the person in line with the magnetic direction of the earth and the soul of the dying person is believed to leave the body with less pain and agony.

It is a custom among the Hindus that when the death of any person is impending and is feared any moment, the patient is laid down on the earth to breath his last. This custom prevails according to the above belief about the soothing effect of the magnetic currents of the earth on the human bodies.

Magnetism and electricity are two branches of the same natural force. They are inseparable and they go side by side. The earth is not only a huge magnet but a vast electrical reservoir too, as an electric current, when released, finds its way into the earth. The human body also is a miniature form of the earth. There is exchange of matters, magnetism and electricity in human bodies. That is the reason why improvement in health occurs by walking on dewy grass or by sleeping out-doors on newly mown hay. The Yogis believe that in some mysterious way the power enters their body and restores energy.

Magnetism in the other Astral Bodies

We have so far considered the magnetism of the earth. If

we go a little further, we find that not only the earth, but the whole universe is permeated with magnetism. As the earth is profoundly affected by the attractive emanations of the sun and the moon, these are dealt with separately in a little detail.

The Sun

The sun is a large natural magnet and has great attractive power. It is attracting all other planets which remain revolving around it under its magnetic influence.

The earth is especially related to the sun. It rotates on its axis and also revolves around the sun. The rotation causes days and nights and the revolution causes years. During revolution there are great changes on the earth due to different exposures of its surface to the sun's rays. These changes make seasons and consequently influence human beings in many ways.

The sun represents fire while the moon rules water. Heat, light and moistures are necessary for all kinds of growth. As the sun and the moon provide these requirements, they help a great deal in production of all eatable and vegetation as well as in the maintenance of life on the earth.

The Moon

The moon too is a great natural magnet. Both the dark and bright fortnights of the moon have great influence on our lives. Many things of our routine life are affected by the moon. The ancient Indian calendars were made with reference to the moon. The dates of women's menstrual periods are counted with reference to the lunar calendar. The time and date of observance of many festivals in the Hindus as well as in the Muslims are determined with reference to the appearance of the moon.

The moon through its attractive force, causes tidal waves in the seas. Similarly, the human bodies which consist of about seventy per cent of liquids are greatly influenced by the moon. Statistics have proved that body fluids flow more freely at the time of full moon. It has also been established that the lunatics get their worst attacks on full-moon days. The word 'lunatics' has been derived from the word 'Luna' which means moon.

The custom of fasting on new-moon and on full-moon days has been considered highly scientific, since it helps in reducing the body fluids and in maintaining proper equilibrium in the body.

Many diseases as well as medicines are also affected by the magnetic effect of the moon. Some diseases are aggravated in the days of full-moon and some medicines work better when administered on full-moon days.

There is a certain Ayurvedic medicine for *Asthma* which is given to the asthmatic patients on the night of the *Sharad Poornima* (full-moon night) which generally falls in the month of October each year. That medicine is taken with *kheer* in the early hours of the morning, after keeping the *kheer* openly exposed to the especially effective rays of the moon throughout that night. The same medicine works better if taken that night in that way, due to the special magnetic effect of the moon-rays on that night. This shows how an important role is played by the magnetic force of the moon on our health and lives.

Similarly, other planets also have their magnetic effect on our lives. Such effect of the different planets together with that of the sun and the moon, forms the basis of astrological calculations and predictions.

Thus we find that all the planets in space have their magnetic powers and give out astral emanations, like the terrestrial objects. They exert their influence upon each other as well as upon every organised being, including human beings, in proportion to their size, their distance and the velocity of their revolutions.

The strength of the magnetic field of the Earth is approximately 0.5 *oersted* while that of the Sun is 25 to 50 *oersted i.e.*, 50—100 times greater.

It is thus clear that the earth, the sun, the moon and all other planets have great magnetic influence on our lives.

Part II

4

Effect of Magnetism on Living Organism

General Influence on Living Beings

Let us now direct our studies to ascertaining the effect of magnetism on living organism—namely, on the worlds of (*i*) Plant life, (*ii*) Animal life, and (*iii*) Human life.

Man seems to have been fascinated by the mysterious powers of a magnetic field over life since ancient times, but a true scientific study of its effect on living matter was not made until the first quarter of this century. It is during the recent period of about the past fifty years or so that a considerable research and investigational work has been carried out in different countries to observe and record the effect of magnetism on living organism. It is during this period that several reports on the effect of magnetic field on life—from bacteria to animals have appeared from time to time and several studies have been published in various journals and books. However, only little is still known about the extent of the effects of magnetism on human beings and still further less about its therapeutic effect in the cure of the diseases of the human beings.

It has been noted that the nature of the magnetism of the huge natural magnet 'the Earth' and that of the small man-made magnets whether electromagnets or permanent magnets is the same except that the intensity of their magnetic power differs. The effect of the magnetic fields is regular and continuous. The constant flow of energy emanating from the magnets, either from the big natural magnets or from the small artificial magnets, connot be interrupted or stopped according to our wish and it continues to have its influence on all the objects within its field as long as the objects remain in its field.

A magnetic field is created by a magnet within the bounds of its effect on all the biological systems of plant, animals and human beings. In the case of the magnetism of the earth, it contributes to the propagation, growth and sustenance of life on its surface. There is a great possibility of extending the life span of all living creatures and also of bringing about complete cure of many sufferings of human beings, by the use of magnets as remedial agents if magnetotherpy can be fully developed.

The question of the power of the magnet or the magnitude of the magnetism to be used in each case is very important. Hence a problem to be considered in any experiment is about the strength of energy that is to be applied. As far as plants are concerned, a solution to this problem seems to lie in treating seeds with magnetic fields. By exposing seeds for different lengths of time to a known strength of a magnet or by increasing or decreasing the strength, the exact point of the full effects of magnets can be ascertained. Thus the needed strength for production of the biggest and the best plants can be fixed. Similarly, experiments on animals and human beings may also be carried out to ascertain what strength of magnetism will be appropriate to obtain the best results.

Dr. Madeleine F. Barnothy, Professor of Physics, College of Pharmacy, University of Illinois, USA, has compiled and edited two volumes of a highly technical book on Biomagnetism. The book is entitled, "Biological Effects of Magnetic Fields" and includes many articles contributed by several scientists of the United States and various other countries such as England, France, Russia and Sweden. Biomagnetism has been defined therein as the 'Science of processes and functions in living organism induced by the static magnetic field'. Reports regarding the results of thousands of experiments of magnetism carried out on mice and other specimens such as bacteria, birds, drosophila flies, fish, molds, pigeons and rabbits as well as on plants and tissue cultures have been recorded in the book.

The experiments referred to above, were made in different ways by many scientists. A large number of experiments was made by exposing mice to as high a magnetic field as 1,20,000 Oe. The mice not only survived these high exposures from 10 minutes to one hour without showing any ill effects, but also improved in weight and remained in good health even long after the exposures. A two-hour exposure of *Neurospora crassia conidia* to a 1,40,000 Oe field, too, produced no mutants.

The results of these studies have valuable implications on the exposure of man to strong magnetic fields. The fact that a mammal survived prolonged exposure to a magnetic field of 1,20,000 Oe increases confidence in the safety range in human exposure. It has been reported that no harmful effects were observed in men exposed to magnetic fields up to 20,000 Oe for a duration of 15 minutes.

Important Conclusions

Some of the other important conclusions arrived at as a result of the experiments are as under :

(a) Magnetically susceptible nutriments such as iron, manganese and cobalt are present in plants in low concentrations as 'trace' elements. They play important regulatory roles in seedling growth.

(b) Magnetism affects every cell in the body of the organism on account of its highly pervasive character.

(c) A magnetic field can exert, without participation of the sense organ, direct influence on the diencephalon (middle brain controlling the endocrine system).

(d) The structure of the forebrain and diencephalon, deprived of any nervous connections with the receptors, react to a static magnetic field more often, more rapidly and more intensely than an intact brain.

(e) Magnetic treatment has a stabilising effect on the genetic code.

(*f*) A consistent and noticeable effect is produced by magnetic field on healing of the wounds. Pathologists have confirmed that fibroblast proliferation and fibrosis are reduced in magnetic fields. Microscopic evaluation also revealed a marked reduction in fibrosis due to magnetic treatment.

The author of that book has expressed the hope that magnetic field will in due time develop into a powerful new analytic and therapeutic tool of medicine.

Dr. Howard D. Stangle of New York, USA, believes that Magnetism is a true science and has observed that this is a subject that should excite universal interest. In fact many experiments have already been carried out in several countries of the world including India. The experiments have been made in different directions with different view-points and have naturally led to various conclusions. It has, however, been noticed that biological effcts are influenced by both the magnitude of the field and the duration of exposure. The results of some important experiments made in various countries are given below :

Results of Experiments in USA

(*i*)   The representatives of :

(*a*) West Virginia University,

(*b*) University of Illinois, and

(*c*) Biomagnetic Research Foundation have, after extensive investigations, concluded that there is a change in the position of the bacteria due to the influence of a magnetic field. This change is on account of their inherent motion.

(*ii*) The department of Biological Sciences, North Western University have observed that there remains no reasonable doubt that living systems are extraordinarily sensitive to magnetic fields.

(*iii*) The Medical Science Department, AVCO Corporation, Willington, Massachusetts, have affirmed that, under favourable circumstances, static magnetic fields can produce observable effects on models which are representative of living tissues.

(*iv*) An eminent professor of Orthopaedic Surgery, State University of New York, opines that there is little doubt that some interaction exists between the function of the Central Nervous System and external magnetic fields.

(*v*) The division of Biology and Experimental Medicine Cincinnati, Ohio, has declared that the results of the study of various types of cells indicate that both the qualitative and quantitative effects of a magnetic field are visible on tissues of respiration and are correlated with several biological factors. It can be concluded that a magnetic field has an effect on cellular metabolism which is related to the type and age of the tissue and that this effect is correlated with the strength of the magnetic field.

(*vi*) Dr. Hansan has stated in a clinical report that a constant magnetic field reduced the sensation of pain.

(*vii*) George N. Cotham of the National Aeronautics and Space Administration, Washington, D.C., relates :

"Careful and precise studies of magnetism and its effect may open up a new approach to biology since the entire body is an electrical organism basically ; from the characteristic electrical charge and valences of atoms of bioelectric energy in nerves. organs and tissues. Fields of magnetic energy properly applied and directed might, therefore, affect the electrical response behaviour pattern. It has been ascertained that the heart rhythmically beating motivated by an electrical impulse produces a very minute magnetic field".

(*viii*) Other experiments were also conducted which indicated the influence of a magnetic field on ageing.

Results of Experiments in Russia

(*i*)   The Institute of Physiology of Academy of Sciences, Azarbaijan, USSR, have studied the effect of a constant magnetic field on the blood picture as well as its effect on the Erythrocyte Sedimentation Rate (ESR). Conclusions have been arrived at, on a detailed study, that there were changes in the blood picture resulting from exposure of the organism to a constant magnetic field.

This information may prove useful to physicians in the diagnosis of diseases of the vascular system as well as of other systems.

(*ii*)   The Institute of Higher Nervous Activity and Neurophysiology, USSR Academy of Science, conducted various experiments on several fish nnd rabbits and arrived at the following conclusions :

(*a*)   A magnetic field is a weak stimulus. The reaction to this stimulus takes place approximately in 40 to 70 per cent of all cases when magnetic field is applied.

(*b*)   A magnetic field produced predominantly an inhibitory effect.

(*c*)   A reaction to a magnetic field sometimes persists even after the latter is discontinued.

(*d*)   A static magnetic field acts directly on the structure of the diencephalon and forebrain.

In connection with (*a*) above, it may be added here that according to the Arndt-Schulz law of Pharmacological action, "Small stimuli encourage life activity, medium strong stimuli tend to impede it and very strong stimuli are apt to stop or destroy it".

Experiments on Animals

A number of experiments on animals carried out in Russia go to prove that insects, mice, etc. are greatly affected by magnets. Dr. L.V. Komarov, a Biologist at the Institute of

General Genetics and Vice Chairman of a newly formed National Committee on the artificial prolongation of human life, has experimentally doubled the life of houseflies by feeding them magnetised sugar. He has also conducted experiments on human volunteers involving various bio-chemical changes to prolong life beyond 100 years. He is hopeful that humans can live for 400 years by the aid of magnet and magnetism.

Another set of experiments by Russian Scientists aimed at extending the life of a mouse by nearly half of its normal expectancy with the use of a plant and magnetic fields. The treatment included harmones and use of low frequency magnetic fields. One of the mice under experimentation created a surprise by giving birth at the advanced age of four, the normal span of white mice being three years.

Results of Experiments in Japan

Numerous experiments have been made in Japan with different magnetic products manufactured by various companies. Most of the experiments made on the stiffness of shoulders and high blood pressure were carried out with Magnetic Health Bands*. As a result of these experiments, the following comments, observations and conclusions have been made :

Comments

(1) An electromotive force is induced by wearing a Magnetic Health Band ;

(2) The electromotive force created by the Band acts upon all blood vessels passing beneath the spot on which the magnetic band is worn ;

(3) The absolute of electromotive force in itself is small. Hence the living bodies are affected by the action of this force over an extended period of time.

(4) Although the living bodies are affected, the phenomenon which takes place is very complex and the mechanism

*Manufactured by M/s. AIMANTE TRADING CO. Ltd., 3-3, 1-Chome, Nishi Shinjuku-Ku, Tokyo, 160, Japan.

leading to the results manifest in experiments is unknown.

Observations

The undermentioned four factors are believed to govern the extent of the effects brought out by magnetism in living bodies :

(1) Strength of the magnetic field,

(2) Length of time in the magnetic field,

(3) Area of living body penetrated by lines of magnetic force, and

(4) Blood flow velocity.

Conclusions

(1) Magnetism has a definite effect on living bodies.

(2) Magnetism proved of great effect in the treatment of some special ailments, and

(3) The effect of magnetism is due to :

(*i*) The activity of living bodies within the scope of the magnetic field,

(*ii*) The induction of an electromotive force in a portion of the magnetic field, and

(*iii*) The physical changes which occur within the magnetic field.

Dr. Shiro Saito of Jikei Medical College, Japan, has been successful in treating cancer tumours of mice with magnetic treatment and believes that this disease in human beings could also be treated similarly.

The above information and other published literature goes to show that Biomagnetism provides an assuring promise for, and satisfies a long-felt need of, proper knowledge of basic physiological processes and their use in therapeutics. Biomagnetism also provides a new system of treatment of various ailments of animals and human beings on a progressive line.

The foregoing information applies to animated organism generally. Let us now come to the study of the effect of magnetism on the three categories of plant life, animal life and human life separately, with some details.

Experiments in U.K.

Hitherto it was known that a magnet had power of attraction of the metallic iron. However, a recent discovery in UK opens up possibilities of newer areas of the utilisation of the magnetic force. The scientists usually had to resort to a tedious chemical method of separation of R.B.Cs (containing iron-rich haemoglobin from other blood cells and plasma. The recent experiments in UK with the use of magnets for separation of R.B.Cs not only simplifies and hastens the process of separation but also goes to prove the positive effect of the magnetic force on the iron in the chemical form. The brief process is as follows :

The red blood cells may be separated from the other blood components using a high-gradient magnetic separator which is generally used to remove micronsized paramagnetic particles from solutions. The magnetic properties of the red blood cells which enable them to separate from whole blood are : that ferrihaemoglobin (methaemoglobin)—present in R.B.C.'s as 1-2% of all haemoglobin and in larger quantities in some diseased states—has a greater paramagnetic susceptibility than the ferrous form (5), corresponding to five uncoupled electrons. Red blood cells are flexible biconcave discoid bodies and occupy approximately 45-50% by volume of whole blood. Haemoglobin molecules carry out the respiratory functions associated with blood and these molecules occupy some 28% of the volume of each R.B.C. The magnetic susceptibility of red blood cells is estimated to be 3.88×10^{-6} when the haemoglobin is under completely deoxygenated state.

In the high-gradient magnetic separation technique, the red blood cells which contain 4% iron are magnetically attracted to a very simple form of steel wool filter. The standard magnetic field of 17.5 kilogauss was used and the magnetic field gradient close to the wires was estimated. The device has been made from very simple components *i.e.* on electromagnet and stainless steel wire filter that can be easily sterilised and made compact and cheap. The device can be adapted to continuous flow processing which is otherwise not possible with conventional centrifugation. A typical high-gradient magnetic separator device consists of a pad of steel wool in a magnetic field which because of small dimensions of its strands introduces a very large field gradient, attracts the red blood cells to the wire and holds them back while other blood components pass freely through. When the magnet is switched off, the steel wool gets demagnetised and the red blood cells can be washed off in a separate container.

Presently, the blood components are separated by placing the blood in a tube and spinning it at a high speed in a centrifuge. However, this method is not suitable in case where pure red cells or white cells are needed.

Effect of Magnetism on Plant Life

Loius Pasteur discovered in 1862 that the earth's magnetic field exercised a positive effect on the growth of plants. It hastened the growth of all plants.

Dr. Noak, the Director of the Institute for Plant Physiology in Berlin made the following observation :

"Electrical measurements of the plant body have shown us that, indeed, electric currents influence decisively not only the absorption of water and nutrient salts, but also other life processes, including the division of the cell".

This is very much similar to the remarks of an Austrian Chemist, Baron Von Reichenbach, after he had experimented with magnets, ten years earlier.

It has been demonstrated by some horticulturists that under the influence of the South Pole of a Bar Magnet, green tomatoes ripen much faster than others only a little away from such an influence. The effect of natural and artificial magnetism on seeds, plants and trees is being further studied by the biologists.

In 1960, some Russian scientists found that the seeds sown in the ground with their tips turned towards the south germinated long before the others. In order to further confirm the results, the buds of wheat, maize and pea seeds were put in facing either the north or the south magnetic poles of the earth. The plants with seed buds facing the south magnetic pole grew with such vigour that the correctness of the earlier result was substantiated beyond doubt. Thus certain claims made centuries ago were confirmed. Artificial magnetic fields were also found to exercise the same effect on the growth of plants.

A number of experiments carried out in many countries have produced other promising results, such as plant fertility can be increased, their tissues can be rejuvenated and protection from frost can be provided by the use of magnets. These factors and many others are capable of enriching the subject of gardening and agriculture with entirely new concepts.

It has been found that low density magnetic fields do not harm the seeds in any way. On the other hand, they provide active help in rapid sprouting and growth and ultimately result in better yields. But plants should not be exposed to magnetic influence for longer periods as in such cases the result could be reversed.

Sometimes, the plants under magnetic fields do not show better growth above the earth but they develop deeper with widespread roots under the earth.

Dr. Fujiyama of Japan has observed that crops sown under the high voltage power cables showed extraordinary growth and vitality in comparison to the crops sown in other places. They were also found greener than the others.

In the 'Soviet Land' Magazine of October 1970, an article showing the potentialities of magnetised water has been published. It has established that plants irrigated with magnetised water grew 20 to 40 per cent faster than others.

Dr. R.S. Thacker of Delhi also has experience of better growth of flower plants through the use of magnetised water. Whenever he felt that some flower plants were drying up, he applied magnetised water to their roots and noticed that only one dose kept them alive for a long time.

Effect of Magnetism on Animal Life

Dr. Harold S. Alexander of North America has observed that if the mice are treated with magnets, they lose malignancy and increase their life span by 45 per cent than the untreated ones. This increase in the life span is achieved by exposing the mice to magnetic field for 6 weeks. He is also of the opinion that the magnetic field has effect on the rate of cellular reproduction of animals.

Dr. Bhattacharya of Naihati Centre, West Bengal, implanted cancer tissues in mice and rabbits. He discovered that after being exposed to magnetic field, the development of cancer in them was controlled and stopped. The cancer tissues were repeatedly implanted in the same mice and rabbits but they were repeatedly controlled by magnetic treatment. It has thus been established that magnetic fields are useful for control of cancer and other types of affections. Moreover, he concluded that the magnets prolonged the lives of these animals.

Experiments have also been made with eggs. Fresh eggs were kept exposed to magnetic fields of small magnets for varying periods ranging from 30 minutes to 5 hours. It was found that the eggs treated for about 30 minutes hatched out one or two days earlier, while eggs exposed to magnetic field for longer periods did not hatch out earlier but, on the other hand, produced smaller chicks. It shows that longer exposure gave reverse results. In some other experiments. magnets were kept inside the cages of chicks. It was found that chickens instinctively came running to the magnets for getting comfort and strength, but did not stay near the magnets for more than 5 to 7 minutes. The chicks paid no attention to dummy models substituted for the magnets.

The female mice kept in the magnetic field of South Pole suffered lesser pains before the delivery and gave birth with comparative ease than the mice kept in the magnetic field of the North Pole.

A mouse, after a life of one-and-a-quarter year, starts showing signs of old age and dies after a few months. If a mouse, in the period of his old age, is treated with a magnetic field of 3000 or 4000 gauss twice a day for one hour at a time in the morning and in the evening, all its ageing symptoms disappear and it looks only 6 or 8 months old.

A horse-shoe magnet of 3000 gauss was used to control the cancer in the mice. For increasing its life, either pole of a 2500-gauss magnet was used.

A dog had a tumour in its brain. It could not walk with its hind legs. The North Pole of a small magnet was tied to the dog's head for five minutes, every morning and evening. This cured the dog of the tumour and it started walking and even running in a week's time.

A Japanese Director of T.I.K.E.I. Medical College successfully treated the cancer tumour of mice with magnetic treatment. He had the faith that similar treatment could benefit human cancer also.

Effect of Magnetism on Human Life

Dr. E.K. Maclean, a New York City Gynaecologist, treats the cases of advanced cancer with an Electromagnetic Activator. He has achieved remarkable success although he has treated only those cases which were considered hopeless.

Dr. Maclean has claimed that cancer cannot exist in a strong magnetic field. If the deadly cancer cannot exist, no other ailment from which a human being can suffer, can exist too.

The high magnetic fields provided by Dr. Maclean to his patients, have also produced a pleasant side effect in restoration of pigmentation in the hair of his patients. In a number of cases, the colour of the hair changed from silvery white to the original natural colour.

Dr. Maclean has dark brown hair on his head. He is tall and robust and at the age of 64 looks to be of about 45 years. He has been applying a 3600-gauss magnetic field to himself daily for a number of years.

Dr. Maclean has succeeded in relieving pains due to any cause by applying magnets.

Almost all human diseases have been successfully treated through magnets in India as well as in other countries. Different cases successfully treated with magnets have been quoted in another chapter of this book.

Not only magnets but even magnetised water has been found to have very favourably acted upon the human diseases and has worked as a beneficial medicine in many cases. Patients with stones in kidney and gall bladder were especially treated by magnetised water in a Leningrad Clinic in Russia and it helped to wash out the salts and stones from their organisms. The magnetised water has special effect on digestive, nervous and urinary systems of man.

Dr. Bhattacharya has quoted wonderful effects of magnets in his book "Magnet and Magnetic Fields". He narrates a very interesting fact. He once visited a factory manufacturing magnets of all sizes and powers. The senior worker in the factory told him that all his married male colleagues had begotten only male children, after their joining the factory. Dr. Bhattacharya calls upon the experts to investigate in the matter. The contact with magnets could indeed be a boon to many people not yet blessed with male children.

These are some examples of the effects of magnets on the human beings. These examples prove that magnetotherapy can be equally useful and effective and in some cases even better than other medical systems. Extensive researches should, therefore, be made in this field and this therapy should be developed for the treatment of even the supposedly incurable cases of mal-functioning of the various systems working in the body.   ★

5

Human Magnetism

Ancient Philosophy

The whole universe, comprising infinite galaxies of stars, planets and all-pervading cosmic consciousness, is delicately balanced by magnetism. The man being a tiny iota of the macrocosm, also carries similar elements, similar properties and similar qualities as the great universe. He is a tiny universe in his own self. In the whole gamut of evolution, starting from the development of five fundamental elements through the unicellular structures and early plant and animal life up to the present man, the latter shares all the subtle as well as crude forces of the universe. Hence the structure of man must also be balanced by the same magnetism which preserves and keeps together the earth, the other planets and the whole universe.

Human existence may be regarded as a trinary entity consisting of three components, namely, body, mind and soul. Man's mind and his spiritual tendencies indicate the presence of a magnetic force, which varies in intensity and effect depending on the subtlety and purity of the inner self. This statement has been amply verified and proved in the practice of the ancient sages and yogis in India. Since time immemorial, the yogis have been concentrating for the sake of purification and enlightenment of mind and soul through a process of meditation. Their miraculous powers of healing by merely extending a touch or a blessing are too well-known and need no description or explanation. Through constant spiritual practices and attempts at the purification of mind, through high thinking and truthful living, every cell of their body is permeated with subtle magnetic powers, which work upon a sick man by a mere touch or by a spoken word. And they can lead to cure. Innumerable instances of such cures through a pinch of *Vibhuti* (Ash) from the hands of the elevated souls are cited in many books on religion. In such cases, the 'magnetised' *Vibhuti* works on the diseased body and alleviates the sufferings. Such yogis are but the high-power human magnets which attract the sufferers around.

Magnetic Powers of Great Personalities

The well-known instances of Swami Ramakrishna Paramhansa and his disciple Vivekananda throw considerable light on the magnetic powers of the master. A light touch of Ramakrishna Paramhansa on the body of Vivekananda transmitted such a strong magnetic current into the latter that he had to cry that he could not bear the forceful power and that the whole place seemed revolving.

Similarly, Lakshman, the brother of Sri Rama, created such a strong magnetic field by drawing a line in front of the hut of Sita that the powerful Ravana could not break through it with all his gigantic powers.

To quote another similar instance, we may recall that Guru Nanakdevji was once sitting along with a few of his disciples at the foot of a hill. Suddenly a scoffer on the hill pushed a huge boulder down the hill to crush the resting guru. The guruji almost instantly pointed his hand towards the boulder to stop it and provided a strong magnetic prop to it. And to the wonder of his disciples, the boulder stopped midway on the slope of the hill—an unbelievable phenomenon.

Another instance : Maharshi Dayanandji, Founder of Arya Samaj, was once travelling in Upper Hill areas on a religious mission. He was climbing a high hill. Just then a very strong storm arose. Maharishiji stopped walking, stood firmly and raising his left arm shouted at the storm, "O Storm, I say you must stop now." And the storm stopped immediately. This was one of the feats of the personal magnetic power of the Swamiji.

Let us now consider some instances from the Holy Bible :

(*i*) Once a leper came and prayed to Jesus Christ to cure

his leprosy. Christ extended his hand and touched him, and immediately his leprosy was cleansed.

(*ii*) A certain ruler came to Jesus and said, "My daughter is even now dead, but come and lay thy hand upon her and she shall live". Jesus arose and followed him to his house. When he saw that his people were crying, he said to them, "Give place, for the maid is not dead, but sleepeth". They laughed him to scorn, but when they gave him way, Jesus went in the house and took her by the hand and the maid got up.

(*iii*) Once two blind men followed Jesus Christ crying and saying, "Thou have mercy on us." He touched their eyes, saying "According to your faith, be it unto you". And their eyes were opened.

Many books on religion of different faiths are replete with such instances and go to speak of the manifestation of the amazing magnetic powers exhibited by many great personalities.

It is a custom amongst the Hindus that people touch the feet of the saints, gurus and elderly persons. The latter bless the former by placing their hands on their heads. There is a scientific reason behind such a practice. It helps in imbibing favourable magnetic force of the realised souls and the elders by the minds and bodies of the youngsters, making them pure and strong.

Personal Magnetism

It is noticed that certain persons, men and women, possess a higher dynamic and magnetic personality and people are spontaneously drawn towards them.This is entirely due to the enhanced magnetism in their person. Such extraordinary powers of magnetic attractions are sometimes their inborn natural qualities or divine gifts and sometimes personal achievements resulting from wilful attempts through practice of some exercises. The natural factors that go a long way to give a person magnetic charm could be both outer and inner. Under natural physical factors may be counted attractive features ;

clear complexion, and a vital, energetic body; while total or partial absence of complexes in thought and expression ; one's healthy *sanskaras* spontaneously leading to enlightened way of living ; high human values ; and intellectual, artistic and spiritual tendencies and faculties constitute the inner magnetism gifted by God. Deliberate and wilful pursuits for attaining higher mental and spiritual power would, of course, go a long way in cultivating and developing the inborn attributes and even in creating fresh possibilities.

It is often noticed, in routine dealings, that positive or negative responses and reactions in certain persons are so spontaneous, strong, beyond our grip and sometimes seemingly maniacal that they leave us agape. This phenomenon of human magnetism can only be explained in terms of attraction or repulsion.

From the days of yore, man has tried to examine and understand this phenomenon of human magnetism and substantiate the same with scientific experiments and explanations. The early experiences of man remained limited mainly to some mystic powers and hence the science or the art was restricted to very few persons with spiritual urges and inclinations who could imagine and visualise the awesome cosmic currents to a limited extent. Amongst these, some of the notable persons of European origin in the recent times, are Paracelsus, Mesmer, Gassner, Hall, Freud, and so on.

Mesmer and his Mesmerism

The art of acquiring, arousing, developing and utilising human magnetism was raised to its peak by Dr. Mesmer. To perpetuate his name, the art he practised and advocated was named Mesmerism. Mesmerism and hypnotism paved the way for the advanced medical science by utilising them in psychiatry. A short history of the art of development of human magnetism and the allied occult sciences is given below :

Dr. Franz Anton Mesmer (1734—1815) was the pioneer of the promotion of the art of human magnetism. Born in Switzerland, he studied medicine in Vienna and developed the convincing idea that a man is influenced by some forces from the other parts of the universe, which effected him strongly. His doctoral thesis was entitled, "The Influence. of the Planets on the Human Body' which was in accordance with his belief about astral effect.

Dr. Mesmer was influenced by the theories taught and advocated by a famous Swiss Alchemist, Physician and Mystic, Phillipus Aureolus Paracelsus (1493—1541 A.D.), who travelled Europe, Asia and Africa for making new discoveries. Paracelsus propounded many new theories and brought a revolutionary change in the minds of the sixteenth century physicians by declaring that minerals such as iron, mercury and sulphur offered better cures for the sick than the then used roots, herbs and plants. He believed that the curative powers of minerals lay in the power of their magnetism as they inherited these properties from the heavenly bodies. Thus Paracelsus gave out that a magnet contains medicinal powers and can be used as an effective medicine. He strongly believed that by passing a magnetic force over the diseased organ, cure of various ailments could be brought about through its magnetic powers. Mesmer was further influenced by the practice of Father Hall, the Jesuit Professor of Astronomy and Court Astronomer to the Empress of Austria, who treated nervous men and women by applying magnets to their bodies as remedial tools. Mesmer had closely watched Hall's work and was greatly struck by the details of responses given by his patients. Deeply inspired, Mesmer decided to take up study of magnets and to use them on his patients. He experienced wonders in their use.

To quote an instance, Mesmer treated the case of a lady, named Franzl Oesterline aged 29 years, by applying magnets. She complained of suffering from periodical spells of severe headache followed by delirium, vomiting associated with paroxysms of rage. No medicine could cure her. Mesmer applied his therapy with three magnets to her body—two over each of her legs and the third on her stomach. As soon as the magnets touched her body, she began to twist her body with pain and convulsions. This condition lasted for a few minutes and thereafter she told Mesmer that she felt as if currents had charged through her body. She was amazed to declare that her pains had gone while previously the attacks lasted for hours together. Next day she was again struck with the same trouble and Mesmer gave the same magnetic treatment again. This time she remained free from her troubles for a longer period. After a few more treatments, her attacks disappeared completely. This gave Mesmer much encouragement and he started using magnets on many patients, for the cure of their diseases and disorders.

Mesmer came in contact with Dr. J.J. Gassner, who posed mysterious motions with his hands while staring into the eyes of his patients. Gassner's technique was to achieve the same cure with his touch of fingers as Mesmer got with his magnets. Mesmer thought over the position, searched for an explanation and concluded that the effects he had produced with magnets could be obtained by his hand too. So he discarded his magnets and followed the procedure adopted by Gassner. He achieved great success by this method also. The number of his patients so increased that he could not cope with the load of work. Thus his new method of treatment became widely known as mesmerism. The doctors of the contemporary age, specially of the conventional medicine, could not accept the theory and the art of his mesmerism, yet unhappy, nervous, physically-ill men and women used to gather in large number at his mansion as patients for treatment and help.

Dr. Samuel Hahnemann (1755-1843), Founder and Master of Homoeopathy, who was a contemporary of Mesmer, confirmed the existence of the dynamic force in mineral magnets after careful experimentation, and advocated the use of the two different poles of the magnet. He also confirmed the effectiveness of Animal Magnetism (Mesmerism) and observed that it is a marvellous, priceless gift of God to mankind, by means of which the strong will of a well-intentioned person upon a sick one by contact and even without contact, can bring the vital energy of the healthy mesmeriser endowed with this power into another person dynamically (just as one of the poles of a powerful magnetic rod upon a bar steel).

Magnetism, Psychoanalysis and Psychiatry

Many others followed the practice of Dr. Mesmer or contributed their own ideas about the technique of mesmerism and hypnotism. Of these, important ones are Pinel, Charcot. Brever and Freud. Sigmund Freud (1856—1939) qualified as a doctor in Vienna but abandoned general practice of the conventional medicine and devoted his life entirely to the treatment of nervous diseases. He was the first to stress that thoughts, desires and cravings are sometimes suppressed and locked up in the planes of unconscious and to show that if these conflicts and complexes could be brought to the conscious level, successful treatment could be effected. He observed that the dreams offered opportunity for release of suppressed feelings and provided important clues and sources of psychic treatment for ill-health. He wrote a book "The Interpretation of Dreams", which was published in the year 1900, and explained therein the mysteries of dreams. The conclusion reached and theories propounded in this book made him famous far and wide. The works of the philosophers mentioned above show how discoveries concerning mesmerism, hypnotism and psychoanalysis were made and how they had impact on medicine.

The medicos never gave recognition to mesmerism and hypnotism, perhaps for fear of losing their thriving business. They have remained unconvinced of these mystic and seemingly fantic methods. But the importance of unconscious mind is being increasingly appreciated now by the medical profession and we find more and more physicians adopting psychoanalytical ways of treatment and even becoming whole-time psychiarists. There are psychiatric services in almost all hospitals, all over the world at present. Simultaneously, more and more physicians are also recognising the effect of magnetism in the treatment of patients and magnetotherapy is gaining ground in many advanced countries of the world, namely, America, Russia, Japan, Denmark, Norway, Switzerland and the United Kingdom. In India also, a number of physicians are doing good service to the sick community by the use of magnets as described in subsequent chapters.

6
Human Body—An Automatic Machine with Magnetic Properties

Brain and Heart Most Important Parts

The human body is a very complicated and wonderfully automatic machinery and its internal functioning is like that of an electric machine. The brain is the controlling switchboard for the whole body mechanism. The nervous system as well as the other systems working in the body are regulated through different controlling centres in the brain. In the circulatory system, the heart works as an electrical generator, supplying energy to the entire body through circulation of blood. Thus the brain and the heart are the most important parts of the human machinery. Let us, therefore, make specific study regarding the functions of these two important organs.

Human Brain and its Functions

The human brain (Latin—Cerebrum, Greek—Encephalon) is a highly organised apparatus. It is a wonderfully intelligent, active and natural centre that controls the functioning of the organs of vision, hearing and speech as well as the motor and sensory nerves. The brain acting through nerves, controls the muscles all over, including those of the face, joints, and neck as well as vagus which stretches into the heart, lungs, intestines, kidneys, liver and spleen. The brain is the centre that receives, digests and gives meaning to man's experiences, initiates and regulates thoughts, emotions and actions whether of conscious or of unconscious origin. The machinery that holds 'MIND' is responsible for our joys, delights, laughter, smile, dancing and singing as well as for our sorrows, griefs, despondency, lamentations, fears, terrors, etc.

The brain consists of nearly 10 billion nerve cells or neurons. Each neuron has a white, thread-like fibre extending from either end and each such fibre interconnects multiples of fibres from one or more other nerve cells. Sensations are conveyed to the brain along the tiny nerve fibres and when they reach the brain, certain electrical impulses are caused by means of which messages are sent to the limbs. These are all electrical effects.

The brain shows not only evidence of electrical activity going on within but also generates small currents which cause 'Brain Waves'. These waves may normally appear at a frequency of about 10 per second, but they often vary in their frequency and size. This variation differs from man to man. In fact, each individual differs in the pattern of his brain waves. The waves transmitted direct to the hands cause a distinctive difference in handwritings.

The force that upkeeps the functioning of the machine works like electricity. In a man, whether asleep or awake, sane or insane, an average adult-size brain generates and operates about 20 Watts of electric energy. The source of the electricity is the individual nerve cells, each of which is in effect a tiny dynamo. From a chemical fuel of glucose and hydrogen, the cell generates within itself an electric charge, and when the charge exceeds a certain level, the cell discharges. As a rule, the greater the stimulus (from danger, emotions, etc.), the greater the rate of charge and discharge. If more adjoining cells fire, the result is a sensation, a pain, a stimulant thought or a feeling of a specific kind.

The nervous system, through which outward sensations are carried to the mind, is so mysteriously built that if we could look inside this system, it would appear like crowded highways, in big cities, especially on the days of week ends.

Electro-shock Therapy, which generally passes 100 to 200 volts of AC current through a patient's head for a mere instant, has been a great help to psychiatrists in treating certain varieties of mental disorders, especially deep depression. The electro-

encephalograph (EEG) by means of highly sensitive receivers
held against the scalp, and radio tubes, which amplify the
faint impulses they pick up, makes it possible to record the
electrical activity going on in the various parts of the brain. In
taking an electroencephalograph, electrodes are applied to the
skin of the various parts of the outer head. The resultant complex curve (EEG) of a human being shows various rhythms.
The character of these rhythms varies with the functional state
of the brain, namely, rest, activity, sleep, etc., and with certain
diseases, namely, brain tumours, cerebral haemorrhages, epilepsy, etc. Thus an EEG is not only a method of determining
the functional state of nerve cells of the brain but also helps
to establish the character of disease in some cases.

The complex structure of the brain normally weighs about
1300 grams in an adult.

The functions of the brain, according to Ayurveda, can be
summarized as follows :

(1) It is a place of *atma* (soul).
(2) The centre of *chetana* (consciousness).
(3) The seat of *panchendriyam* (special senses).
(4) Store house of *buddhi, medha* (intellect).
(5) The seat of *chitta* (consciousness).
(6) Store house of *smriti* (memory).
(7) Centre of *jiwana* (life).
(8) Regulator of *nidra* (sleep).
(9) Seat of *rajas* (emotion, passion).
(10) Centre of *snayu* (nerve centre).

Human Heart and its Functions

Now let us study the make up of the heart (Cor or Cardia).
The heart is made up of thousands of muscles which may be
taken as the composing elements. It consists of two complex
systems of cells—one constituting the auricles and the other
ventricles—which are again divided into two parts each. The
details of the structure of heart have been given in a subsequent
chapter. Here we may concern ourselves with the mechanical
and electrical side of its working. Taking a graph of the

functioning of the heart is technically called Electrocardiography (ECG). In taking an electrocardiogram each chamber is considered separately. Each mechanical contraction, auricular or ventricular, is associated with two electrical processes. The first is depolarisation, during which process the electrical charges on the surface of the muscle cell change from positive to negative ; the second is repolarisation, which follows the first and results in the return to the resting state and replacement of the positive surface charges. Depolarisation is a rapid process whereas repolarisation is slow.

Muscular activity of the heart is associated with electrical activity. It is the electrical phenomenon of the heart muscles which produces the electrocardiogram. No current is recorded unless contraction of the heart muscle occurs, with its associated change in the membrane permeability.

The electrical activity of each element of the heart can be measured by a vector—a force which may be represented by magnitude, direction and sense. The sum total of vectors may be considered to be the resultant vector of the electrical activity in the entire heart.

The heart generates electrical energy and breathing has a close connection with the beating of the heart. If the breathing could be controlled, the action of the heart too could be controlled, and by allowing periodical rest to the ever-acting heart through the art of control over breathing, life could be prolonged indefinitely. The way to slow down the process of the electrical discharge and subsequent decay of the body is to bring about a change in the process of quick metabolism. The practice of *yoga* teaches this art. It is quite well-known that *yogis* in India generally go to the Himalayas to practise the art of *yoga* in a cool and silent atmosphere. Sometimes they fall into trance, suspend all animation, for some indefinite periods, remain motionless as if at complete rest and recharge their discharged batteries. Then after some time, they revive themselves and thus defy the ravages of time.

To make a more serious study of the action of the heart, we may refer to the innumerable positions which the heart may assume as demonstrated by Ashmon's description of 45 different Electrocardiographic positions. For clinical purposes, however, only the following six positions of the heart may be noted :

    (1) Horizontal position.
    (2) Semi-horizontal position.
    (3) Intermediate position.
    (4) Semi-vertical position.
    (5) Vertical position.
    (6) Indeterminable position.

The blood circulatory system originating from the heart is also a very complicated mechanism. The heart is a strong and tough muscular compact located at the mid-centre in the body. It may, however, have a break-down like all other machineries. There may be many reasons for the break-down of the machanism of the heart or its constituents. When any part of the heart machinery is impaired, the part of the body affected does not receive the blood supply it needs and is damaged. The damage may occur in heart itself or in any-other related part of the machinery, namely, brain, lungs, kidneys, limbs or skin.

The chemicals of which the body is comprised, namely, carbon, nitrogen, oxygen, phosphorus, etc., combine to form a perfect electric battery, and the food we eat enables it to charge itself. The body too, therefore, exhibits its electrical responses.

The electrical potential of the stomach varies when it goes empty and becomes full, in sickness and in health.

It has been observed that when blood sugar runs low, electrical changes take place in the brain. Normally, recording of the waves reads from 8 to 10 cycles a second, but when the concentration of sugar in blood is lowered, this rate drops to 5 or 6 cycles per second.

The electrical activity functioning in the system of a living human being has the capacity to generate electricity within itself for its full requirement. The human body may, therefore, be taken as an electrical battery. It is capable of emanating electromagnetic waves at the rate of 80 million cycles per second, which is beyond the perception of our visual capacity. Every human body is constantly discharging static emanations which may be taken to represent either electricity or magnetism. To quote an instance, every human being can act as an aerial to receive powerful wireless signals by putting one's hand on the aerial socket. It has also been noticed that keeping a hand on a transistor and placing it in North-South direction gives clearer and better sound.

A battery needs chemicals for its composition ; we need food and drinks to work as battery. By means of some mysterious alchemy, these chemicals generate the electric current that replenishes the battery.

Spiritual powers cannot exist in the presence of unholy things. Therefore, unholy desires, wrong thinking and faulty living can destory the means of regeneration and do a great harm to ourselves. Usually, ill-health and sometimes even death is caused by demolition and disintegration of the cells consequent upon faulty energy. When faulty energy is put into action, it turns things wrong towards evil thinking, opposing good thoughts.

There is a common belief that electricity is the cause of life. Innumerable experiments have been conducted and electrical fields have heen found to exist in the most elementary form of embryo. It has accordingly been proved that the body of every human being contains some element of electricity and some properties of associated magnetism right from the beginning to the end of life.

Magnetic Fields in Human Body

Today's scientists and medical specialists have proved that the human body is a source of magnetic field. Attempts have been made to measure the magnetic fields produced by different organs of the human body, namely, heart, brain, nerves, muscles and other tissues as well as the frequency of magnetic fields in some diseases. It has been found that the magnetic fields,produced by all the organs in the body that consist or contain muscles and nerves,is of fluctuating nature.

Astoundingly, the peak value of the fluctuating magnetic field produced by heart is greater than 10^6 gauss. Similarly, some muscles when flexed produce high frequency magnetic fields whose **peak** value is 10^7 gauss. It has been found that the strongest magnetic field from the nerve tissue is from brain which produces its largest fields during sleep. It has an amplitude of 3×10^8 gauss. In certain diseases like epilepsy larger fields can be produced.

The source of magnetic fields in human body has been ascribed either to the presence of sodium, potassium, chlorine ions that the nerves and muscles generate in the process of contraction or signal transmission. This has led to measurement of the magnetocardiogram and magnetoencephalogram for measuring the ion currents of the heart and brain respectively. Another possible source of magnetism in the body is the presence of magnetic materials.

Besides the fluctuating magnetic fields produced by different organs, there are steady magnetic fields. Because the strength of earth's steady magnetic field is about 0.5 gauss, the steady fields from the body are to be measured in a steady background that is greater by four or more orders of magnetic amplitude. The measurement of current flow for fluctuating magnetic field is done in terms of (A.C.) and steady current as (D.C.).

Some of the advantages of measurement of magnetic fields of heart, brain, lungs and other organs may be to evaluate the condition of an organ and to know any impending malfunction or defect. For instance, the magnetocardiogram may be used to investigate heart when it is injured by the curtailment of blood supply. Some of the conditions like, Ischemia, associated with this type of trouble can be detected in time and further complications like angina or infarction,avoided.

The use of magnet in various diseases including those connected with the brain and the heart has been dealt with separately in a relevant chapter.

7

Role of Blood in Human Body

The scope of this treatise is to study the therapeutic effects of magnetic power on human ailments. The magnetic force works on the human body through the circulatory system. Hence the knowledge of the functions of the blood, the heart and the circulatory system are very important for this method of treatment. Let us, therefore, note some details about them before we proceed to discuss the principles, methods and technology of the magnetic treatment.

The blood is a fluid that circulates through the heart, arteries, capillaries and veins carrying nourishment and oxygen to the tissues of the body and taking away waste matter and carban dioxide from them.

Composition of Blood

The human blood is composed mostly of a fluid part called plasma in which red corpuscles, white corpuscles and platelets are suspended. Blood consists of 78 per cent of such fluid and 22 per cent of solids. The details of the constituents of blood are as follows :

$$
\text{Human Blood} \quad
\left.\begin{array}{ll}
\text{Water fluid} & 78\% \\
\text{Solids} & 22\%
\end{array}\right\}
$$

The break-up of the solids is as under :

Proteins	=18.5 per cent
Salts (Inorganic)	=1.5 per cent
Lipids (Fats)	=1.4 per cent
Glucose	=0.1 per cent
Waste products	=0.5 per cent

A. Cells   (*i*) Red blood corpuscles (Erythrocytes)
                45 to 50 lacs per cubic millimetre.
           (*ii*) White blood corpuscles (Leucocytes)
                5,000 to 10,000 per cubic millimetre.
          (*iii*) Platelets (Thrombocytes)
                2 to 5 lacs per cubic millimetre.

All these cells are very minute, remain floating about in the liquid and are visible only under the microscope.

B. Fluid Plasma—This is comprised of the following
            ingredients :

(1) Water—(90-92 per cent of total fluid).
(2) Gases—Oxygen, carban dioxide, nitrogen.
(3) Foods—Carbohydrates (glucose), fat (fatty acids),
        Protein (amino acids).
(4) Blood Proteins—Serum albumin, serum globulin,
        fibrinogen,
(5) Salts— (*i*) Chlorides of sodium.
            (*ii*) Bicarbonates of calcium.
           (*iii*) Sulphates of potassium.
            (*iv*) Phosphates of magnesium.
(6) Protective substances—Agglutinin. antitoxin, bac-
            teriolysins, opsonins.
(7) Autacoids—Internal secretions from ductless glands.
(8) Waste—Urea, uric acid, creatinine, xanthine, hypo-
        xanthine, gaunine, adenine, and carnine.

The blood is a red, non-transparent, nutritive fluid and has a peculiar odour. Arterial blood is bright red or scarlet and the venous blood is dark red or crimson. It is of alkaline reaction and is salty in taste. Its specfic gravity is 1050 to 1060. The body of a healthy adult contains about 5-6 litres of blood, which weighs about one-thirteenth or one-fourteenth of the total body weight.

The red blood cells (erythrocytes) contain a protein pigment, called Haemoglobin, which provides red colour to the blood. Iron is one of the main constituents of the haemoglobin.

Haemoglobin readily unites with oxygen and just as readily gives it up. When blood in lungs gets saturated with oxygen, all the oxygen combines with haemoglobin of the red cells, but when the blood passes into the distant organs where oxygen has already been used up by the cells, the haemoglobin gives up its oxygen to the cells. The oxygen content in a human adult averages from 12 to 17 pet cent (12-17 grams of haemoglobin in 100 grams of blood). The red blood cells are so small that a line of 3000 of them would fall a little short of 25 mm in length. The human body contains about 25×10^{12} (25,000,000,000,000) red cells.

The red blood cells are small disc-like bags, 8 mm in diameter, occupying 45 to 50 per cent of the total blood volume. They are flexible biconcave discoid bodies. Haemoglobin molecules occupy some 28% of volume of each red blood corpuscle.

A molecule of haemoglobin has approximately 10,000 atoms. of which 4 are iron. The iron atoms are essential for respiration process and they give the blood its characteristic red colour. These atoms contain enough iron to make the red blood cells weakly paramagnetic so that they are influenced by magnetic fields.

The white blood cells (leucocytes) vary in size, are actively mobile and change their numbers and shapes. They perform a protective function. They engulf and destroy bacteria and discharge enzymes and other substances into the blood plasma, which help to fight the infectious agents that might have entered the organism.

The Platelets (thrombocytes) are very small and irregularly shaped structures, They contain a substance called 'Thrombokinase' which participates in blood clotting.

The red blood cells as well as the white cells die and disintegrate in blood. New corpuscles are continually being produced by bone marrow in the organism to replace the dead ones. The rate of their death and reproduction is estimated to be about 10,00,000 a second. There are about 500 to 800 **red**

corpuscles for each white cell. When the number of red blood
cells falls too short or the red cells do not contain enough of
haemoglobin, the body fails to procure proper amount of
oxygen and to maintain its level of energy. This causes diseases like anaemia. Since haemoglobin is a protein substance,
foods rich in protein are essentially needed to balance our daily
diet.

The blood plasma is a viscous, lightly yellowish, protein
fluid. The cellular elements of the blood are suspended in
the plasma. It consists of 90-92 per cent water and 8-10
per cent organic and inorganic substances. The plasma is
closely linked with the tissue fluids of the organism. It contains
a special substance, called 'Antibodies', which plays a protective
role. Some of them are able to neutralise toxins, others destroy
the bacterial growth which might have found a way into the
organism.

Blood Circulation

The process of continuous flow of blood in the organism is
called the system of blood circulation. All the organs of a
living human body are in close communication with each other
through the circulation of blood. The heart pumps the blood
so as to reach even the distant extremity of the body. The
activity of the system of circulation is modified by the nervous
and respiratory systems.

The blood flows through the blood vessels, which are elastic
tubes of varying diameters. The blood vessels too differ among
themselves in structure and in function. The blood flows, so
to say, through a sealed circuit of vessels about 1,12,000 kilometres in overall length, most of which is occupied by capillaries. The blood travels through the arteries at a speed of more
than 65 kilometres an hour, but it takes a minute for the blood
to go through 25 mm of capillary tube.

There are three main types of blood vessels, namely,
Arteries, Capillaries and Veins.

Arteries are vessels through which the blood flows from the
heart to various organs. They have comparatively thick walls

made of three coats. They divide into smaller branches, called Arterioles, which again divide into still smaller vessels called capillaries.

Capillaries are minute blood vessels visible only under a microscope. There are several hundreds of capillaries per square milimetre of tissue of the organs. It is through these minute capillaries that the blood, oxygen and chemicals reach the smallest and the remotest part of the body and waste products are collected from there. As the blood flows through a capillary, the arterial blood changes into venous blood, which drains off into the veins.

Veins are vessels through which the flow of blood is carried back from the organs to the heart. Like those of the arteries, veins too have walls composed of three coats. Veins contain valves which open in the direction of the blood flow. This helps the blood in the veins to flow in the direction of the heart.

Clotting of Blood

The blood possesses the property to clot, that is, to change into a thickened mass of blood. Normally, the blood flows through the blood vessels freely but sometimes blood clots are formed and they obstruct its easy flow. Such a clotting or sudden blocking of passage is technically called thrombosis (formation of thrombi). The blood usually clots after escaping from the blood vessels. The human blood escaping from the organism clots within 3 to 4 minutes.

Sometimes, the arteries are clogged with a deposit of fat, calcium or cholesterol. This also can obstruct the flow in the smaller arteries. Then sometimes the inner coating of the vessel gets roughened and if the blood clings, clots may be formed building up obstruction in the blood stream or forming a blockade in the vessels of the heart or brain. If a clot gets into any of the arteries carrying blood into the brain and cuts off the oxygen supply, the brain cells die. If the victim escapes, the damage to the particular part of the brain may cause rupture, cerebral haemorrhage or paralysis. However, this property of clotting has some advantages too. The clot stops the opening of an injured vessel and further bleeding is stopped. If clots did not form when blood flowed out of a vessel, the slightest wound would cause bleeding without stoppage.

Sometimes, progressive degeneration spreads to the muscular coat and the elastic tissue is replaced by fibrous tissue, and sometimes deposits of calcium salts are formed in a way that the flexible tube becomes an intractable pipe. This is called hardening of the arteries or arteriosclerosis. When this hardening or thickening affects the main arteries, additional demands are made on the heart and consequently the heart has to increase its pressure. The additional effort of the heart to maintain blood circulation is called high blood pressure. Serious high blood pressure or systematic hypertension may be due to some other causes as well.

Heart (Cor or Cardia)

The heart is a hollow, muscular, cone-shaped organ located in the anterior cavity of chest. The greater part of the heart is situated in the left half of the thorax. The heart is about the size of an adult person's fist and weighs about 300 grams. The wall of the heart consists of three coats, inner or endocardium, middle or myocardium and outer or epicardium. The entire heart is enveloped in membranous sac called pericardium.

The human heart has four chambers. A longitudinal partition divides it into right and left halves. Venous blood flows through the right half and the arterial blood through the left. Each half of the heart consists of two chambers, the upper called the Atrium and the lower called the Ventricle. The wall of each atrium forms a projection in front called an auricle

Vessels entering and leaving the heart—The two largest veins, which carry the venous blood from all parts of the body empty into the right atrium. The largest arterial vessel, the aorta, which carries arterial blood for the entire organism, arises from the left ventricle. The heart is supplied with blood through the right and left coronary arteries, which arise from the aorta.

The heart is a very strong and tough bundle of muscles and works very hard all the time. It has to be so as it is to pump blood for a whole lifetime, without stopping for repairs. It is, therefore, necessary that it should receive an uninterrupted supply of oxygen and nutrients. In the course of an average life time, the heart beats 1250 million times. Even the toughest metallic machinery could not endure if operated incessantly for, say, seventy years.

Action of Heart

The work of the heart consists of rhythmic contractions and relaxations of the atria and ventricles. You can get a rough idea of the action of the heart if you clench your fist, open it, and then clench and open it again. If you open and close your fist, again and again, at a rate of a little more than once every second (as the heart beats), your muscles will feel tired after a couple of minutes. Our heart is, however, contracting and dilating at an average rate of 72 times a minute, which adds up to over 1,00,000 times a day or nearly 40,000,000 times a year. The only rest the heart muscles get is the fraction of a second pause between beats.

A contraction of the heart muscle that squeezes out the blood from the chamber is called a Systole, and the subsequent relaxation of the heart is called a Diastole. The contractions and relaxations of the heart take place in a definite order. There are three phases of cardioactivity :

Phase   I—Simultaneous contraction of both atria, with the blood passing from the atria into the ventricles.

Phase   II—Simultaneous contraction of both ventricles, the blood is forced into the aorta and the pulmonary trunk, while the atria relax.

Phase III—The ventricles relax and the atria are also relaxed. This is called the general pause. During this pause, blood enters the atria from the venous vessels.

Thus the systole of the atria is followed by the systole of the ventricles and then by a pause. All these three phases constitute a single cycle of the heart-action.

Atrial systole lasts about 0.1 second, ventricle systole 0.3 second and the pause 0.4 second. Thus one complete cycle of the heart action takes about 0.8 second, so there are about 75 contractions of the heart per minute. At rest, the number of contractions ranges from 60 to 80 per minute but the rate and intensity of the cardial contractions vary with environmental conditions, namely, physical exertion, etc. The heart rate also depends on age. In the new-born, the heart contracts about 140 times per minute, and in old age the rate increases up to 90-95 per minute.

Diseases of Heart

The cases of the diseases of heart are increasing, in the highly developed countries, at an alarming rate. In our country also, the rate of the diseases of heart is on the increase. Obviously, it has a lot to do with the pace of life we lead and the stresses and strains of modern life. In the present age of rapidity, resistance and tensions, which we call modern living, we are surely supercharging the engine of our internal machinery, namely, the heart.

The term 'heart disease' applies to a number of different illnesses that affect the circulatory system. It points more to cardiovascular disease – cardio (heart) and vascular (blood vessel) or the disease of circulatory system.

Some people are of the opinion that most of the cardiac ailments result from excessive smoking, emotional strain, high blood pressure, diabetes, fats, obesity, excessive use of salt and even excess of sugar. A certain degeneration in the circulatory system gradually takes place as people grow old and the arteries are hardened as a result of the build-up of fatty substances on the inner walls of the blood vessels. This naturally reduces the speed of flow and passage of blood to and from the heart, causing cardiac trouble.

Usually by a 'heart attack' is meant what is generally called coronary thrombosis (myocardial infarction). It is a sudden blocking of one of the arteries that supply the heart muscle with blood. A clogged artery may be closed by a blood clot (thrombus) and the part of the heart muscle fed by that artery may deteriorate or die from lack of blood.

Another common complaint is 'Angina Pectoris'. It is an uncomfortable sensation of pressure, tightness or pain usually in the front of chest. It indicates that the heart muscles are not getting enough oxygen through its blood supply. An attack may be the result of over-exertion, excitement or over-eating. The pain of Angina starts over the breast bone and radiates down the inner side of the left arm sometimes down both arms, and into the middle fingers. Every time a person with this condition exerts himself in an effort for which the heart arteries cannot supply sufficient blood, this pain warns him and compels him to stop further exertion. This happens over and over again until he learns to lead his life in a lower gear. Nature gives this warning to pull him up to lead a regulated life before his heart muscle is dangerously affected or causes shortage of oxygen.

The human blood is divided into four groups. Hence, for the purpose of transfusion, the blood of donors and recipients is matched before transfusion and only compatible blood is transfued to the bodies of the recipients.

Blood Pressure

Normally, the blood pressure is constant ; and if it varies, the variation is negligible.

Changes in blood pressure depend on two basic factors, nemely : (*i*) the force with which the blood is ejected from the heart by the contraction of its muscles, and (*ii*) the resistance of the walls of the blood vessels, which the blood has to overcome as it circulates in the body.

The blood pressure is usually measured in the brachial artery. In a healthy young adult (20-40 years) of our country, the maximal pressure in this artery is 110-130 mm and the minimal is 60-80 mm. In children, the blood pressure is lower but, in elderly people, the blood pressure slightly increases. During physical work also, blood pressure rises but it drops during rest and sleep.

In diseases associated with disturbances in blood circulation, the blood pressure is altered. In some cases, it is elevated and is called hypertension or high blood pressure and in some others it is lowered, when it is called hypotension or low blood pressure. Hypotension may be caused by a decrease in the number and intensity of the cardiac contractions, dilation of the arteries and considerable loss of blood. A big drop in blood pressure leads to serious disturbances in a human being.

Functions of Blood

The main functions of blood in the body are as follows :

(1) The blood streams carry nutrients to the tissues of all organs. The nutrients are absorbed into the blood from the small intestine.

(2) The blood carries the waste matter away and throws it out of body. The waste products are eliminated from the blood through the excretory organs.

(3) The blood plays a vital role in respiration. It delivers oxygen to the tissues of the organs. Oxygen enters the blood through the lungs.

(4) The blood removes the carbon dioxide from the system. Carbon dioxide is eliminated from the blood mainly through the lungs.

(5) The blood regulates the activities of the natural fluids of various parts of the body. It transports various hormones round the organism. Some of these substances stimulate, while others initiate the work of the organs.

(6) The blood has a protective action. It contains cells which possess special products called antibodies, which play a protective role.

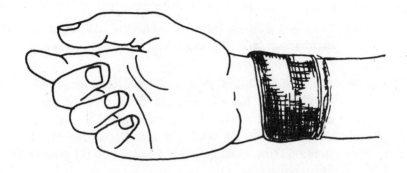

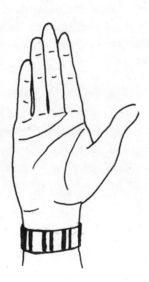

Blood-Circulation (B.P.) Belt: For reducing high blood pressure. Tie the Belt on right wrist and for increasing low blood pressure apply the same belt on left wrist.

(7) The blood distributes heat within the organism and maintains a constant body temperature. The heat is transported by blood from warmer parts of the body to the cooler parts.

(8) The blood gives off the excess of heat into the external environment and the organism, therefore, does not become overheated.

(9) A part of the blood does not circulate through the blood vessels but is stored in small blood depots, namely: capillaries of the spleen, liver and tissues. In the case of muscular work and blood loss, the blood stored in the small depots is released into the general blood circulation.

(10) The total amount of blood may temporarily increase after intake of large amount of liquids and absorption of water from the intestines. The excess water is quickly eliminated through the kidneys, while a temporary decrease in blood is sometimes observed by way of bleeding.

If the Blood Stops Circulating, the Organism dies

We have seen here the important functions carried out by blood in our bodies. We shall discuss in the subsequent chapter, how magnets, when brought in contact with the body, affect the blood and exercise their beneficial influence on all the diseases of the human body, through the blood circulatory system.

Part III

8

How Magnets Affect Human Metabolism

Different Theories of Biological Effects

We have seen in the previous chapter that blood plays an important role in the human body. Anything which affects the blood, either favourably or adversely, is sure to have a good or bad effect on our health. Let us now study the mode of influence of magnets on the blood and consequently upon human health and life.

Magnetism is a physical phenomenon as well as a phenomenon closely related to electricity. It is not easy to comprehend a phenomenon like magnetic field theoretically. Hence it may be difficult for those who are specialised in biology and medicine, to fully appreciate this phenomenon but the fact remains that it has its biological effect on human beings.

A magnet not only attracts iron and several other things but it has other qualities also not known to every one. One of these qualities is that the magnet also attracts all martial humours that are there in the human system.

Martial means (iron—Pertaining to or containing iron) (Humours means any fluid or semi-fluid substance in the body).

In ancient medicine, the four juices, namely: blood, phlegm, black bile and yellow bile of which the body was thought to be composed, were called humours. The magnet, therefore, is very useful in all inflammations, influxes and in ulcerations, in diseases of the bowels and uterus, and in internal as well as external diseases.

Various theories of biological effects of magnetic fields on human beings have been propounded. It is considered that the biological effects of magnetic fields depend on many factors such as flux density, directivity, gradient, area of magnetic field affecting the living body, duration of its action, etc. The effects of magnetic fields on the living body are ascribed to several factors, such as :

(*i*) the possible occurrence of the impediment in the microbial movement and protoplasmic flow resulting from their motion in the direction at right angle with the magnetic field,

(*ii*) action against the growth of the young tissue (action against mitose),

(*iii*) influence on the human autonomous nervous system,

(*iv*) magnetohydrodynamic phenomenon, and

(*v*) reciprocal difference in the magnetic susceptibility.

The Most Popular Theory

The most popular theory offered so far is that the effect originates in the molecules containing iron such as haemoglobin and cytochromes. These theories are proposed because of the well-known paramagnetic properties of iron. A few of these theories are briefly described below :

(A) (*i*) Scientists of several countries discovered, in the earlier part of this century, that the process of crystallization in solutions is influenced by magnetic fields. It was proved, on the basis of a large number of experiments, that the magnetic field increased the number of centres of crystallization.

One of the scientists has summarised the effect of magnetic field on liquids as follows:

(*a*) a magnetic field increases the number of crystallization centres in a liquid,

(*b*) the increase in the amount of crystallization centres is directly proportional to the strength of the magnetic field, (*c*) in the case of constant field, the number of crystallization centres increases directly with the time of imposition of the magnetic field.

(*ii*) It was established, as a result of many experiments and experiences, that many physical and chemical properties of water change when it is exposed to the influence of weak magnetic field. The change takes place in its various properties and the changed properties exist for a long time, namely, its temperature, density, electrical conductivity, surface tension and viscosity.

(*iii*) It was also noticed that if a vessel containing water is enclosed in a metal cover which can absorb the electromagnetic waves, it immediately affects the speed of sedimentation of tiny particles in water.

The blood is also a fluid and is, therefore, similarly influenced by magnetic fields and its properties also undergo a change when it is brought in contact with magnets.

(B) When a fluid in which salt is dissolved comes in contact with magnetic flux, the physical properties of the fluid change. As blood is a fluid matter and many inorganic salts form its important constituents, the properties of blood change under magnetic flux. This changed blood coursing through the whole body exerts beneficial · influence on the entire body and relieves or prevents many ailments.

(C) When a magnet is brought in contact with the human body, a weak electric current is generated in the blood circulating in the body. When the weak current runs through the blood, the quantity of ions is increased and the ionised blood circulates throughout the body, with good effect on the body as a whole.

Action of Magnetic Flux on Blood

The clinical studies conducted by many medical institutions have shown that the magnetic flux promotes health and provides energy by eliminating disorders in the various systems working in the body, stimulating blood circulation and building new cells to rejuvenate the tissues of the body. The magnetic flux greatly affects magnetic substances like iron and oxygen with the result that the haemoglobin in the blood vessels moves actively to effect the activated circulation. The treatment with magnets increases the number of new sound blood corpuscles. The ratio between the red blood corpuscles and the white blood corpuscles is not disturbed but inactive and decayed blood corpuscles are appropriately strengthened and more fresh vital blood is pumped into the system. As magnetic power promotes better breathing action also, it results in prevention and cure of the diseases connected with circulatory system *i.e.*, bronchitis and asthma. According to a clinical study, high blood pressure comes down by 20-30 mm Hg by using magnets for a week or two.

Action on Hormone Secretion

The function of internal secretion of hormones is remarkably improved by the joint effect of internal heat of the body and the external heat caused by the magnet. The transmission of blood is done rapidly against this heat and the capillary vessels, which spread like a net around hormone secretion tubes, expand to a large extent and by concentrating oxygen, they gradually supply hormone secretion into the tubes. Meanwhile, the hormone secretion tubes get properly warm and their function becomes active by supply of excess oxygen. Consequently, all diseases caused by the lack of hormone secretion are favourably affected and improved by the constant use of magnets. While the magnetic flux penetrates the tissues, it works to regulate hormone secretion which preserves youth by providing energy and by normalising the functions of the internal organs.

Pituitary Gland Regulates Height

There is a Pituitary gland—a ductless body—located at the base of the brain. The small reddish gland remains in the sella turcica (depression of the bone) and is always discharging hormone secretion. The secretion governs the body and its growth. If the secretion is normal, the height remains normal ;

if the secretion is more, the height becomes more than usual. If, however, the secretion is less, the height of the person remains less than normal.

Short height is awkward looking and is often a stumbling block at the time of marriage—specially of girls.

Magnets can help such boys and girls to increase their height to some extent up to the age of 14-15 years in normal cases. It may also be tried as a special case, above that age limit if circumstances are favourable. Along with magnetic treatment, some Homoeopathic medicines and physical exercises can also help to increase the height up to a certain age (20-22 yrs).

Reformation and Resuscitation of Cells

The remarkable feature of the power of magnets is seen in the matter of reformation, resuscitation and promotion of the growth of cells. The magnetic flux generates a comfortable warm feeling in the body. The warmth strengthens the function of cells and cures inflammations and spasms. When the magnetic flux passes through a tissue, a secondary current is created around the magnetic lines of force in the tissue cells which ionises the protoplasm and rejuvenates the tissues by activating the metabolism. Consequently, remarkable curative effects have been noticed on human body. Chaps. chilblains and incised wounds have healed up promptly through the treatment with magnets.

Acceleration of Self-Curative Powers

The human body itself cures most of its own diseases. An efficient doctor or an excellent remedy only assists the natural curative powers of the body. The magnetic flux is also a natural healing power and it invigorates the self-healing property of the human body. Strong magnetic flux penetrates deeply into muscles, fatty tissues and bones to give intense relief to the nerves. It enables the body to resist diseases and to accelerate recovery from sickness and fatigue. The collective therapeutic effect of magnets cures diseases by eliminating the constitutional weakness. Thus the curative powers of the magnet do not operate individually or independently but work together and an alround healing is effected, namely, of blood, nerves, hormones, etc.

The use of magnet helps to improve, in a short period, even inveterate diseases. Many cases, which have defied other systems of treatment, have responded satisfactorily to the treatment through magnets. A large number of disorders like appendicitis, asthma, backache, chronic arthritis, cramps, eczema, headaches, high blood pressure, injuries, mental fatigue, orchitis, pains of all kinds, prostate enlargement, rheumatism, severe toothache, sleeplessness, stiffness of joints and swellings of different parts of body have already been effectively cured through this system of treatment. The magnet has a remarkably good effect on the toothache, other pains, swellings, stiffness of joints and muscles and cervical spondylitis which are detailed elsewhere in this book. It also has a good effect on the prevention of, and improvement in, the diseases of the heart, kidneys and liver.

Heart and Geomagnetic Activity

Since time immemorial, effects of geomagnetic activity on the human organism have been known. However, the work on the precise affect of the activity on different organs especially heart has now been carried out. The scientists of the National Geophysics Research Institute, Hyderabad, have recently found a link between the heart attacks and the geomagnetic activity. It is known that the fluctuations in earth's magnetic field are caused by solar flare and sunspot activity. Particles accompanying these solar phenomena reach the earth and generate geomagnetic storms that rapidly alter the earth's magnetic field. The scientists of the above institute observed that heart attack cases "generally occurred during geomagnetic disturbances showing rapid fluctuations and pulsations." These pulsatory fields seem to react with human heart or brain electrical potential and trigger off heart attacks or psychiatric disturbances in persons who are not otherwise in perfect shape and condition. In addition, there are other factors like moon phases (particularly the new-and full-moon), thunder-storms which are responsible for magnetic disturbances

in the atmosphere. It has now been proved beyond doubt
that the electrical potential of the body is normal in bioelectrical
state of the body and its organs are disturbed whenever there
are severe magnetic disturbances in the atmosphere around us—
weaker parts being greatly affected.

In recent years the scientists in Russia have established cor-
relationship of solar and geomagnetic phenomena with cardiovascular cerebral diseases and deaths in a number of towns.
The scientists carried out experiments on the behaviour of dogs
and rabbits under artificial fluctuating electronic magnetic
fields and found that the heart and nervous systems of the
animals were greatly affected. They also observed that the fish
stayed in shallow waters during calm magnetic conditions but
moved off to deep waters when the magnetic activity went up.

Innumerable cases of heart attacks or their perturbed conditions have been reported from all over the world which emphasise
a positive link between the heart attacks and the geomagnetic
activity.

Summary of Beneficial Influence of Magnets

The beneficial influence of magnets may be summed up as
follows :

1. When a magnet is applied to the human body, magnetic
    waves pass through the tissues and secondary currents
    are induced. When these currents clash with magnetic
    waves, they produce impacting heats on the electrons in
    the body cells. The impacting heats are very effective to
    reduce pains and swellings in the muscles, etc.

2. Movement of haemoglobin in blood vessels is accelera-
    ted while calcium and cholesterol deposits in blood are
    decreased. Even the other unwanted materials adhered
    to the inner side of blood vessels, which provoke high
    blood pressure, are decreased and made to vanish. The
    blood is cleansed and circulation is increased. The

activity of the heart eases and fatigue and pains disappear.

3. Functions of autonomic nerves are normalised so that the internal organs controlled by them regain their proper function.

4. Secretion of hormones is promoted with the result that the skin gains lustre, youth is preserved and all ailments due to lack of hormone secretion are relieved and cured.

5. Blood and lymph circulations are activated and, therefore, all nutritions are easily and efficiently carried to every cell of the body. This helps in promoting general metabolism.

6. Magnetic waves penetrate the skin, fatty tissues and bones invigorating the organs. The result is greatly enhanced resistance to disease.

7. The magnetic flux promotes health and provides energy by eliminating disorders, in, and stimulating the functions of, the various systems of the body, namely, the circulatory, nervous, respiratory, digestive and urinary.

8. The magnetic treatment works by reforming, reviving and promoting the growth of cells, rejuvenating the tissues of the body, strengthening the decayed and inactive corpuscles and increasing the number of new sound blood corpuscles.

9. Magnets have exceptional curative effects on certain complaints like toothache, stiffness of shoulders and other joints, pains and swellings, cervical spondylitis, eczema, asthma as well as on chilblains, injuries and wounds.

10. The self-curative faculty (Homoeostasis) of the body is improved and strengthened which ensures all the benefits mentioned above. One feels in full vigour and can walk and work, more and more, without feeling tired.

11. The magnetic treatment has the effect of energising all the systems of the body. The effect remains in the body for several hours after each sitting with the magnets. A continued treatment for a week or two, once daily for about 10 minutes, takes the patient from morbid condition to normal state of health, in general routine cases.

Note : As magnets work on human metabolism mainly through the circulation of blood, which contains haemoglobin and iron, it will be relevant to state the position of iron contained in the body. The adult human body contains 4 to 5 grams of iron and it can be traced in all parts of the body. Most of it is present in blood as a component of haemoglobin and a smaller amount remains in muscles and is called myoglobin. The function of these components is to carry oxygen from the lungs to muscles and other parts. Without iron, there would be no energy ; and without energy, the beating of the heart and respiration would stop. Thus we see that iron is very essential for our life and magnet influences iron radically and magnificently.

✱

9

Magnet and its Composition

Natural Magnets and Artificial Magnets

Magnets may be broadly divided into two groups, namely, Natural magnets and Artificial magnets.

Natural magnets represent the substances created by nature, which have the property of attraction. The biggest natural magnet is the earth itself as shown in an earlier chapter. Some other natural magnets are ironore, magnetite and other iron-pyrites, etc., which contain iron and oxygen and also have the property of attracting iron filings. The force of these natural magnets remains the same and cannot be increased or decreased according to one's wish or requirement. Hence the natural magnets are of very restricted use.

Magnetism was, however, believed to have great power and potentialities, Man has, therefore, made his own magnets and has designed them in many ways to suit his requirements. These man-made magnets are called *Artificial magnets*. The artificial magnets can be made to have different degrees of magnetism and can be manufactured in various designs. These can, therefore, be used for many purposes and are utilised in innumerable items of general nature as well as in cottage and heavy industries.

Electromagnets and Permanent Magnets

The artificial magnets are broadly divided into two main categories, namely : Electromagnets and Permanent magnets.

The electromagnets are magnets which work when electricity is applied to them and have no power of their own to act without electricity. Electromagnets are used in electric machines, generators and motors and are utilised in various industries. These are used for loading and unloading iron-equipment on ships, for magnentic cranes, and magnetic brakes in trams. These are also used for separating iron scraps from other non-magnetic substances, as well as in amplifiers, armatures, bells, buzzers, circuit breakers, contact rectifiers, electronics, loud speakers, reed relays, radios, storage devices, telecommunications, transformers, etc. Electromagnets are also used by surgeons for extracting iron splinters from eyeballs and other parts of body.

Permanent magnets, as their name shows, remain permanently magnetised once they are charged with electric current and are used without electricity applied to them every time they are put to use. They do not lose their magnetism if they are properly preserved with keepers attached to them for many years. If not stocked with keepers, these may, however, lose some force of their magnetism, in due course of time—say in some years, but these can be remagnetised and the decreased force of their strength restored to them. If they are recharged every 5-6 years, they work for 100 years—even more.

Different Shapes, Sizes, Designs and Strength

The permanent magnets are made of different alloys and are of different shapes, sizes, and designs. These also have different magnetic strength. The strength of the magnets depends upon the proportion, quantity and quality of the different metallic alloys which are mixed for making them.

The most commonly manufactured and used shapes and designs of the permanent magnets are given here. The sizes differ according to the requirements and the purposes for which they are made.

1. Bar magnets.
2. Cylindrical solid magnet.
3. Cylindrical magnets with holes.
4. Ring magnets.
5. Rectangular magnets with holes and without holes.
6. Chuck magnets.

7. Arc or Crescent magnents.

8. U-shaped magnents.

9. Horse-shoe magnets.

10. Square magnets with holes or without holes.

11. Cup shape covered magnets.

The above shapes are but examples of the magnets which are generally produced by the manufacturing companies. In fact, permanent magnets can be made, with the alloys already in use, according to any given measurements or specifications to suit any purpose, in any shape, size, design or strength.

Generally permanent magnets are made for industrial, commercial and educational purposes but some of them can be utilised for medical purposes also. They are however of low strength and are not therefore of great use for the purpose of treatment. The author has, after his long experience, developed some special magnets for treatment of chronic diseases. The photos of these pairs of magnets are given at the end of this book.

In some cases, the magnets are attached to the parts of machinery while in some other cases, they are encased in other metallic covers and are then used. When these are so encased, their magnetic power is increased manyfolds. One example of such magnets is the complete magnetic kit or unit prepared for loud speakers. Such magnetic packages are used in many other kinds of machinery also.

Classification of Magnetic Materials

There is a very wide range of magnetic materials from which permanent magnets may be made. The materials differ in the nature of their elements and their composition. Each of them has its own values, its own characteristics and consequently its own uses.

The most commonly used alloy in the manufacture of permanent magnets is Alnico. This is composed of Aluminium, Nickel, Iron and Cobalt. The last of these four metals, namely cobalt, is costlier than the others and Iron is the cheapest of all. As researches have all along tried to make the magnetic material more stable and economical, Alnico alloy has been divided into several standards. The approximate chemical composition of some standards of Alnico is given below :

Name of Metal	General	Alnico II	Alnico III	Alnico V
Al (Aluminium), percent	18	10	12	8
Ni (Nickel), percent	—	20	24	14
Co (Cobalt), percent	12	12	—	24
Cu (Cuprum-copper), percent	6	6	3	3
Fe (Ferrum-iron), percent	64	52	61	51

The different metallic alloys from which magnets are made are called magnetic materials or magnetic substances. The magnetic substances are broadly classified in three main categories, namely :

    (*i*) Ferromagnetic.

    (*ii*) Paramagnetic.

    (*iii*) Diamagnetic.

The general characteristics of these substances are as follows :

(*i*) *Ferromagnetic.* These substances have got very large values of magnetic permeability and are, therefore, capable of high degree of magnetisation. They include the metals which are found to be attracted by magnets or magnetic fields. Such substances are : Iron, Steel, Nickel and Cobalt. The difference between the properties of Iron and Steel is that soft iron has far greater retentivity than steel, but has far less coercivity ; in other words, steel retains magnetism for a long time, whereas soft iron loses it earlier. As such soft iron is used in electromagnets and steel is used for permanent magnets.

(*ii*) *Paramagnetic.* These substances represent the materials which are feebly attracted when placed in a magnetic field. In a non-uniform field, paramagnetic substances will experience an attractive force towards the strongest part of the field. Such substances include Aluminium, Chromium, Copper sulphate, Manganese, Palladium, Platinum, Potassium and Tungsten. etc.

(*iii*) *Diamagnetic.* These substances are the materials which are not attracted by magnets. They have a tendency to move from stronger to weaker parts of magnetic field and are characterised by negative susceptibility. To this class belong Antimony, Bismuth, Copper, Diamond, Gold, Mercury, Silver, Sulphur, Tin and Zinc.

Gases and liquids are also found to belong to the classes of paramagnetic or diamagnetic substances. Air and oxygen are found to be paramagnetic while Alcohol, Hydrogen, Nitrogen and water are diamagnetic in their properties.

Permanent alloy magnets are generally used for door latches, fans, filter coils, gramophones, loud speakers, magnetoes, magnetic generators, magnetic separators, meters, radios, scooters, sugar mills, telephones, television receivers. toy-motors, and other novelties.

Ceramic Magnets

Some magnets are also made from synthetic material and are called ceramic ferrite or graphite magnets. The ceramic or ferrite magnets are manufactured from oxides of Ferric and Barium (or Strontium), with certain doping agents which differ from manufacturer to manufacturer.

Ceramic magnets are used for the purpose of :

(*i*)   Communications—Loud speakers, microphones (bells, inductors, receivers).

(*ii*) Electricals   —Cycle dynamos, D. C. (Small) motors, instruments, toy-motors.

(*iii*) Electronics   —Calculators, computors, tabulators.

(*iv*) Transport   —Car radios, aerial motors, dynamos for autos, magnetoes for motor cycles and scooters.

(*v*)   Miscellaneous   —Belts, door-latches, filters, magnetic-chucks. magnetic-games, magnetic

separators, novelties, plastic materials and stationery items.

Ceramic or Ferrite magnets have the following distinct
advantages :

(1) Considerable higher coercive force and retention of
magnetism for a very long time.

(2) High stability to demagnetising field and temperature
changes.

(3) About 60 per cent weight as compared to metallic
magnets.

(4) Available at lower costs.

(5) No "keepers" necessary for long preservation.

A drawback with the ceramic or ferrite magnets, however, is
that they are liable to break on falling down. Hence they
should be handled with care particularly to avoid chipping of
sharp edges or corners.

Magnets of all types—namely, electro or permanent, iron-
alloys or ceramic—are produced by the manufacturing companies for industrial purposes. There is only one company at
Bombay, Messrs Permanent Magnets Ltd. who make small
Healing Magnets also. The healing magnets are in different
shapes and sizes, are coloured Red, or marked N (North) and
S (South) and are supplied magnetised. The other magnets
supplied by this company as well as other companies for industrial purposes are supplied uncoloured, unmarked and unmagnetised unless a specific request is made for magnetisation.

Magnetisation and Magnetic Poles

After the magnetic materials are transformed into the
required shapes, sizes and designs, the formed pieces have to be
magnetised before they can be put to use.

The magnetisation is done by electric current ; and for
this purpose, electromagnetising machines are used these days,
as they are convenient and powerful. By this magnetisation
process, the formed pieces develop North polarity on one end/

or side and South polarity on the other end or side, in a very
short time, namely, seconds. Magnetisation does not take long
time if one has a "charger" or "magnetiser", and knows how
to operate it.

Established Laws of Magnetism

On the basis of many experiments and experiences, the
following main principles or laws of magnetism have been
established :

1. **Like poles repel each other and unlike poles
   attract each other.** This is a universal rule and it
   can be experienced by any one by taking two magnets
   and bringing one marked pole of one magnet near each
   of the two poles of the other magnet.

2. **Equality of poles of magnets.** As the molecules
   are arranged in lines in the magnetised state of a substance, there are as many like poles on one side of the
   neutral region as on the other. Both the poles of every
   magnet are, therefore, opposite to each other and have
   equal and the same strength. In other words, the pole
   strength at the two ends of a magnet is always equal in
   magnitude but opposite in nature.

3. **Inseparability of Poles.** Every bar magnet has two
   different poles, at its two ends, and so has every other
   type of magnet. If a bar magnet is actually cut into two
   parts, each part becomes an independent magnet having
   two opposite poles like the original one. If the smaller
   magnets be subdivided further, still shorter magnets are
   formed, each having two poles again.

4. **Retention of Magnetisation.** Long bar magnets
   retain their magnetism longer than short bar magnets,
   on account of less demagnetising action of the poles on
   themselves. Horse-shoe magnets and U-shape magnets
   retain their magnetisation longer than bar magnets. And
   magnets with enlarged pole pieces forming closed rings
   encased in round .or square metal cases retain their
   magnetisation still longer and become more powerful.

5. **Demagnetisation and remagnetisation of magnets.** When a magnet is subjected to rough handling (such as hammering, heating or twisting), its strength is impaired, because such treatment partially breaks down the linear arrangement of molecules. Demagnetised magnets can, however, be remagnetised or recharged to regain their lost strength.

6. **Safe custody of magnets.** In order to avoid the automatic demagnetising effect of the poles, magnets are kept in pairs with two ends of the pieces of soft iron strips placed across them. These strips are called 'keepers.' The 'keeper' completes the magnetic circuit and hence there are no free poles to lose their strength.

Power of Magnets

The exact power of magnets can be measured by a gauss-meter which is a costly instrument. Hence the power of a magnet is generally estimated by its capacity to lift iron-weight. The more weight a magnet can lift, the more powerful it is considered to be. A child's horse-shoe magnet sold as a toy (which can relieve toothache) is about 300 gauss. The author uses magnets of upto 3000 gauss power to treat chronic diseases.

It is said that first of all bar magnets were made. As the poles of a bar magnets are at the extreme ends of the magnet, which are distantly and oppositely placed, the power of the magnet is not very strong. Then U-shape or Horse-shoe magnets were designed so that both the poles may be close to each other. Such magnets are more powerful and can lift more iron-weight. But there is a gap or open space between the two poles of such magnets. In order to improve upon these magnets also, ring magnets or solid cylindrical magnets were made, so that there is no such gap between the two poles. Such magnets are still more powerful and can lift heavier weights.

Various Qualities of a Magnet

Dr. A.K. Bhattacharya of Naihati, West Bengal has stated in this book "Magnet and Magnetic Fields"—or "Healing by

Magnets" that a magnet is a miniature universe as all the forces operating in the universe are seen operating in this little thing also. He has described innumerable qualities and properties of the magnet and has shown the different properties which each pole of the magnet possesses separately. The qualities appear to have been pointed out keeping in view a bar magnet, but, on principle, they should be true about every other type of magnet too. The main qualities can be summarised in a tabular from as follows :

Quality	*North Pole*	*South Pole*	*Intervening Portion*
1. Magnetic	Attraction	Repulsion	Neutral
2. Characteristic	Positive	Negative	Neutral
3. Effect	Cold	Hot	Neutral
4. General	Love	Hatred	Indifference
5. Atomic	Proton	Electron	Neutron
6. Planets	Mercury, Venus, Moon	Sun, Mars	Jupiter, Saturn
7. Elements	Earth, Water	Fire	Air, Ether
8. Cosmic colours	Green, Indigo, Orange	Red,Yellow	Blue, Violet

The source of permanent energy of a magnet is not clearly known to science uptil now. It is also wonderful how the poles of a magnet, which is a piece of metal without any life, can recognise the friendship or enmity of other poles and adopt infallible behaviour towards them. This shows that the power of recognition inherent in a magnet is divine in character.

It was on account of the concentration of all these qualities in a magnet that many kings and queens and other high dignitaries of the olden times used to wear a magnet on their persons. They believed that wearing a magnet, which had a divine force, maintained vigour of life, arrested ageing, enhanced beauty and saved its wearer from many ailments and troubles.   ★

Part IV

10

Technique of Application of Magnets

Different Poles have Different Effects

The use of magnets is an aid to nature. The application of magnets works as a medicine and restores the body to its natural state in due course. The treatment through magnets has its effect on body mainly through blood circulatory system and also through other systems, namely, digestive, nervous, respiratory and urinary. It also has its use in geriatrics, gyneatrics and pediatrics. There are several methods of application of magnets to the different parts of the body for the treatment of different ailments. The main methods are dealt with in this chapter.

Ancient literature shows that magnets were used for healing purposes in ancient China, Egypt and in other countries. The ancient magnetotherapists could not make out why the magnets failed to show any effect in some cases and even showed adverse effect in some other cases. Experience and experiments since made with application of different poles on different patients have proved that the two poles of the magnet act in different ways when brought in physical contact with human body, have different properties, characteristics and effects. The North Pole has a retarding action, controls the bacterial infection and pus and makes ineffective or even kills the cancer cells. It also relieves, boils, sores, skin rashes, tumours, etc. The South Pole on the other hand, radiates energy, gives warmth and strength to the painful part, increases power of resistence, reduces swelling and draws pain out of the body. The no-effects or adverse effects noticed by some physicians of ancient times might have been due to the application of magnets of low strength or applying them for shorter or longer periods or using incorrect poles or for some other causes.

Magnetism, regardless of how one may look at it, is a form of energy and does affect all the mankind, animals, vegetation and all other living systems on the earth. The researches made in this respect have found that it can be a valuable tool in many professions not just for the sake of mankind, to arrest, control and destroy diseases, improve mental attitude, etc. but it may also alter all concepts of medical approaches to healing the sick.

Mode of Application

Some physicians and scientists are in favour of using one single pole at a time. Sometimes they suggest application of North Pole for 10 minutes and then immediately thereafter South Pole for another 10 minutes like cold and hot packs in Naturopathy. The principle adopted in this book, however, is to use a single pole only where the disease is located in a small portion of the body and to use both the poles when larger parts or whole bodies are affected by any disease. Single pole theory is an old theory while the bipolar application is based on the latest double pole theory of magnetic treatment.

One of the contemporary propounders of the single pole theory, Dr. Albert Roy Davis of USA, generally uses a bar magnet ($15 \times 5 \times 1.25$ cms) for treatment of various ailments. Some of the cases enumerated by him in his book "The Anatomy of Biomagnetism" are brieflly stated below for information :

North Pole (N.P.)

1. Arthritis — Calcium of joints is slowly dissolved by North Pole.

2   Bleeding or haemorrhage—After birth or due to female weak organs.

3. Bleeding of wounds, cuts, bruises due to weak tissues.

4. Boils and Cancers

5. Broken bones, broken joints, fractures—

South Pole on the upper and North Pole on the lower portion ensures best healing.

6. Burns — North Pole on the burnt portion. When the pain is less, South Pole to give strength to the tissue and to form flesh over the burnt part.

7. H.B. Pressure — N.P. under the right ear down the artery.

8. Infection, pus, discharge due to any infection

(N.P. arrests it and nature heals).

9. Kidney infection or stone (even partially lost kidneys may start fuctioning in some cases).

10. Sprains in ankles, back, hips, legs and feet, etc.

11. Teeth and gums — Decaying teeth, infection of gums, swellings, pus deposits.

12. Toothache with bad smell, bleeding & wounds

South Pole (S.P.)

1. All kinds of pains, stiffness and weakness in fore limbs, arms, legs, shoulders, hips, etc.—S.P. encourages & provides strength and life to the limbs.

2. Encourage life in all its forms but makes infection worse.

3. Digestion poor, gas formation—Due to more acidity in stomach.

4. Production of insulin less.

5. Prostate enlargement (Fluid discharge is increased. M.W. every 2 hours or earlier is a *must*).

6. Hair colouring—S.P. improves hair colouring in limited cases of those persons only whose health is good. South Pole for ½ hour on the seat of the person after he/she has gone to bed gives good results.

7. Heart—We should ascertain the actual heart disease as there may be several types of complaints. For weak hearts, weak heart muscles, causing murmurs, reduction of pulse rate, and heart beats—apply South Pole.

8. Neuralgia (Headache)-the causes should be investigated and treated. S.P. works to remove it if applied also below the left side of the stomach, M.W. and diet should be advised.

9. Weak muscles—South Pole for 10 minutes morning and 10 minutes in the evening again.

10. Weakness to walk—South Pole for a week or 10 days provides energy and strength.

In his book, Dr. Albert Roy Davis has given some discussion about the magnetic development in Russia and America. He then writes as follows :

"If we examine carefully, we will find a form of stimulation of the living system by these two separate and different forms of energy (*i.e.* magnetic poles).

Now from the above discussion, we can better understand the effect of each pole of the biomagnet and the combined results of using both poles of the magnet when used together at one and the same time."

With a view to resorting to more rational methodology as well as in view of the above, we have preferred to adopt the system of applying two poles simultaneously and we call it general treatment under double pole theory as per details given hereunder :

The magnetic treatment is generally carried out in two ways : (*i*) Local and (*ii*) General.

Local Treatment

In local treatment, it is not quite necessary to resort to two magnets *i.e.* to apply both the poles together. The selected pole of a magnet is applied to the affected part of the body directly, next to the skin, that is, in close contact with the bare skin, although it can be applied over one or two layers of cloth also, without applying pressure on it. This is done when the ailment is localised in a particular part of the body, say, for example, in the case of a boil, in mumps or in tonsils, and in the case of pain and swelling of a small portion on account of some injury or otherwise. In the case of diseases due to some bacterial action or infection, the north pole should be applied, while in the case of pain and swelling where no infection is suspected, the south pole should be used. Thus the selection of the correct pole of a magnet for spot application on the body is very important in magnetic treatment.

General Treatment

General treatment is given in the case of ailments not centred in any particular part of the body but affecting major portion of the body or extending to wider area or covering the whole body. This requires treatment by two different poles of the magnets of similar shape, size and stength.

The general rule for carrying out general treatment is as follows. If the disease lies in the upper half of the body, that is, in the parts above the navel, magnets should be applied in the palms of both the hands of the patient and if the disease is more in the lower half of the body, that is, in the parts below the navel, then magnets should be applied under the soles of both the feet. In case the disease spreads to the whole body, the treatment may be given alternatively underpalms and under soles on alternate days, that is, one day in both hands and next day under both feet, or in the morning under the hands and in the evening under the soles if treatment is given twice a day. Here, as a general rule, the North pole should be applied to the right hand or foot and the south pole to the left hand or foot.

The ability to tone up and correct human system lies in the palms of hands and soles of feet. Thus the source of health lies in human palms and soles. It is difficult to believe how they work but there is no doubt that they do.

This book is intended to help the average person to return to and enjoy health by natural means. It is to show how to ease routine ailments and promote well-being. It does not authorise every reader to treat people who are severely ill but surely help every one to regulate the different systems working in the body and consequently to enjoy better health.

The human body is very wonderfully constructed and each part of it is connected with other parts of body, directly or indirectly, through blood-circulation and nervous system. The extremities of the body, namely, hands and feet, are directly connected with many other important organs of the body.

The hands, as well as the feet, have many 'Reflexes', which tie up the different portions of the hands and the feet with various other organs. The palmer and the dorsal sides of the hands have different reflexes. The different reflexes have direct links with various regions of the body, but the palm side is tied up to more important organs. The same is the position with the feet. Hence the palms of hands and the soles of feet are used in general magnetic treatment and the effect of the treatment goes to all the parts of the body, through internal connections.

Electericity and Magnetism

It is a matter of common knowledge that electricity and magnetism are correlated. There is a magnetic flux around the lines of electricity and magnetism can produce electricity under certain circumstances. Hence each of them is so inter-linked with the other that it cannot be completely separated.

Electropathy and Magnetotherapy

In Electricity, there are two currents, namely, Positive and Negative, while in Magnetism there are two Poles, namely, North Pole and South Pole. Both the currents of Electricity match with the corresponding Poles of the Magnet. Therefore wherever Positive current is used in Electricity or Electropathy North Pole is applied in Magnetotherapy; and wherever negative current is used in Electricity or Electropathy, South Pole is applied in Magnetotherapy.

In view of the above, Magnetotherapy works on the lines of Electropathy, at least in some respects. The methods followed in Electropathy in some cases can, therefore, be adopted in Magnetotherapy, with certain modifications.

Standard Lead Technique of ECG

Let us understand Standard Lead technique employed in Electrocardiography (ECG) for further study. The parts of the body employed for the purpose of ECG are two fore-arms (or hands) and the left leg (or foot). These may be coupled in any one of three combinations, each of which is called a 'lead'. Each standard lead uses two electrodes and thus the standard ECG is a combination of two tracings. Lead I consists of electrical tracing produced by a combination of the right arm and the left arm electrodes. Lead II stems from the right arm and left leg electrodes; and Lead III from the left leg and left arm electrodes.. A fourth lead occasionally used, was termed as Chest Lead. It was tested at several parts of the body but did not prove satisfactory. Hence the main leads in use are only three—namely, leads I, II and III.

The ECG shows a graphic representation of the electrical forces produced by the heart. The application of magnets works through the blood and acts through the heart. In magnetotherapy, the use of all the three Leads is adopted as our first three methods of application of magnets. In addition, two more methods to cover all positions are adopted. The additional methods are the combination of (*i*) Right hand and Right foot and (*ii*) Right foot and Left Foot. Thus the main methods of application of magnets in general treatment come to five in number. The reverse of Lead II, namely, Left Hand and Right Foot is neither used in ECG nor it need be used in Magnetotherapy, although there is no serious objection to apply magnets to these parts if any case requires this treatment. The relationship of the magnetotherapy methods to the ECG Leads as well as the Poles of magnets to be applied in each method are indicated below :

Five Methods of Application of Magnets

In general treatment, under double pole theory

Magnetotherapy		Electrocardiography	
No. of method to be adopted	*Pole of magnet to be applied*	*Where to be applied*	*Corresponding ECG Lead*
I	North Pole	Right Hand	I
	South Pole	Left Hand	
II	North Pole	Right Hand	II
	South Pole	Left Foot	
III	North Pole	Left Hand	III
	South Pole	Left Foot	
IV	North Pole	Righ Hand	✗
	South Pole	Right Foot	
V	North Pole	Right Foot	✕
	South Pole	Left Foot	✕

Side-wise Application of Magnets

Besides the 5 methods, mentioned above there are three more principles for application of magnets.

We have seen in Chapter 3 that human body itself is a magnet and our bodies are considered to have magnetic sides. According to that view, if we have to apply the magnets on right side and left side of the body, then North Pole should be applied to the right side and South Pole to the left side. Secondly, if magnets have to be applied on the upper and lower sides of the body, North Pole should be applied to upper side and South Pole to the lower side. Thirdly, if the magnets are to be applied to the front and back sides of the body, then North Pole is to be applied on the front side and South Pole on the back side.

All the above rules are meant for general guidance of practitioners. They can deviate from the above rules and exercise their own intelligent decisions according to every case in hand, if some other and better method of application of the magnets is considered more appropriate in any case.

The method of treatment is selected for every patient or disease, according to the nature or place of the ailment. The North Pole or the South Pole of a magnet is to be applied to the right or left side of the body according to the methods selected for treatment as shown above.

Therefore, in case method I is adopted for the treatment of any person, North Pole should be applied to the right palm and the South Pole to the left palm. If method II is chosen, North Pole should be applied to the right palm and the South Pole to the left sole. The application of the Poles in other methods will be made to the parts of body noted against the respective methods.

Thus, no medicine, no injection, no needle-piercing, no pressurising, no massaging, etc. but only placing your palms or soles lightly on the magnets for minutes and Nature works.

Technique of Contact with Magnets

When treatment is to be carried out by the foregoing methods, two round or square magnets, one having North Pole in its centre and the other having South Pole in its centre, are to be used. A wooden bench, chair or stool and a piece of wooden plank about one inch thick, big enough to provide space for both the feet, should be arranged.

For taking treatment by method No. I, the patient should sit on the wooden bench, chair or stool and should keep the

FIVE METHODS OF MAGNETIC TREATMENT

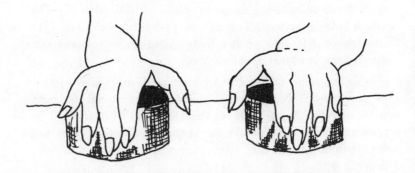

Method-I, North Pole under the palm of the right-hand and South Pole under the palm of the left hand. Used for treating ailments of the upper half of the body, like arthritis of hands.

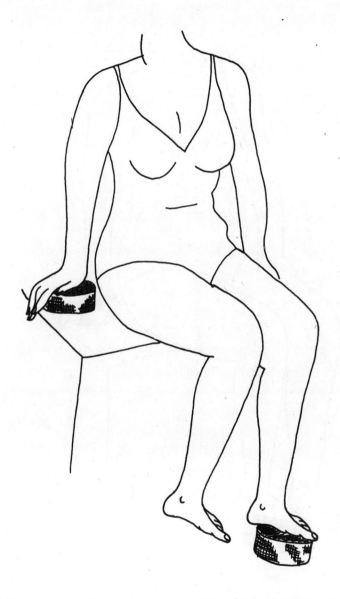

Method-II: North Pole under the palm of the right hand and South Pole under the sole of the left foot. This diagonal application benefits liver, spleen, stomach and intestines. Has a curative effect on the digestive system and cures gastric and other abdomenal troubles.

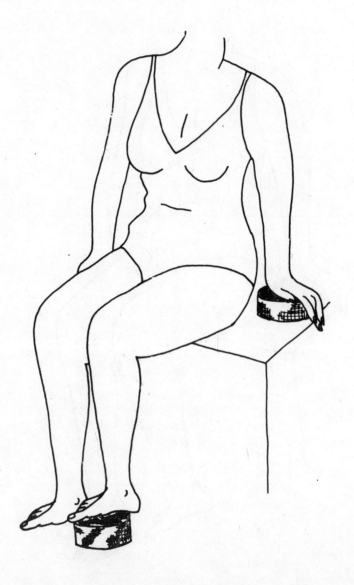

Method-III: North Pole under the palm of the left hand and South Pole under the sole of the left foot. For treating the left-sided ailments like Paralysis, Polio, Pains in left side, general weakness etc.

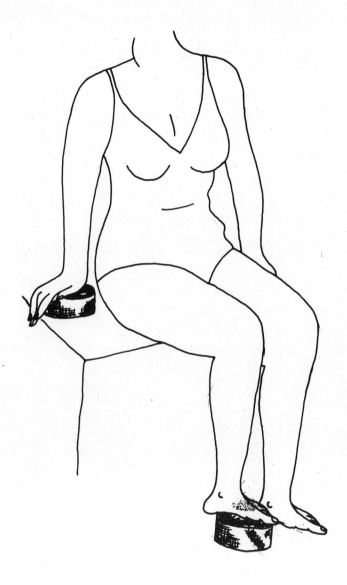

Method IV: North Pole under the palm of the right hand and South Pole under the sole of the right foot, for treating the right-sided ailments like Paralysis, Polio, pains on right side, general weakness etc.

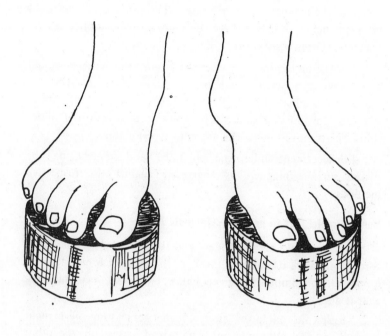

Method-V: North Pole under the sole of the right foot and South Pole under the sole of the left foot, for the ailments of the lower parts of the body, including arthritis of feet and ankles, gout, irregular or low circulation of blood in the legs etc.

magnet having North Pole in the centre on his righ hand side and the magnet having South Pole in the centre on his left hand side. He should then place his right palm on the centre of the magnet kept on his right side and his left palm on the centre of the magnet on his left side. The wooden plank should be kept below his feet. No pressure need be applied on the magnet ; simple constant touching is sufficient.

For taking treatment by method No. V, the patient should sit on a wooden bench, chair or stool, keep both magnets on the wooden plank (North Pole to the right side and South Pole to the left side) and rest his soles on their centres. Shoes should be removed but socks are not objectionable.

For treatment under other methods, hand or feet may be placed on the magnets as suggested against the respective methods.

Some Simple Test to perceive Magnetic Force

Some people may wonder and doubt whether magnetic force can work on, or pass through, the hand or foot placed on a magnet. A simple test, given below, will convince anybody that it does.

"Rest your palm on electromagnet or strong permanent magnet and place a number of small iron pains on the other side (back) of the palm. The pains will stick out like bristles on the back of the palm, proving continuity of the magnetic force through the palm, although the palm itself may not feel any sensation or magnetic effect. This proves that magnetic force not only works on the palm but passes through it and goes beyond". Similarly the magnetic force works in the body through the soles also.

The magnetic force passes through cloth, glass, paper, plastic, rubber, stainless steel and wood too. This can be easily proved by the following tests :

(i) Take any cloth made of cotton, nylon, terelene or wool. Keep some pins on the cloth and pass a magnet below the cloth. The pins will move as the magnet below the cloth is moved.

— (*ii*) Take a glass-tumbler or a steel-tumbler and put some pins in it. Pass a magnet by the side of the outer wall of the tumbler. The pins will move inside the tumbler as the magnet is moved outside. If the magnet is lifted higher than the top of the tumbler, the pins will come out of the tumbler and will stick to the magnet.

(*iii*) Take a hot-water bottle or any thing else made of rubber. Keep some pins on one side and pass a magnet on the other side of the bottle. The pins will move just as the magnet is moved. If the magnet is rotated briskly, the pins will dance.

(*iv*) Take a smooth wooden plank of the thickness of about half-an-inch. Keep some pins on the upper side of the plank and pass a strong magnet under the plank. The pins will move in the direction the magnet is moved.

All these simple tests will prove that the force of magnetism in not checked or stopped by any of the things mentioned above but passes through them.

In fact, whether you touch strong magnets by soles or by palms, the affect of magnetism reaches the whole body upto head. If you go on touching the strong magnets for long periods, you may feel some heaviness, headache, sleepiness, yawning or even giddiness.

Treatment of Diseases

Almost all the diseases where organic or tissue changes have not yet occured, are amenable to magnetic treatment. A list of a hundred and fifty common diseases which can be successfully treated by magnets is given at the end of this Chapter. The appropriate method of application to be adopted in each of these diseases as well as some additional hints have been indicated against each disease for facility of treatment.

Selection of Magnets

The shape, size and design of a magnet is to be selected according to the convenience and suitability of its application to the particular part of the body where it is required to be used. There are parts of body where large-size magnets will not fit in and there are some other places where small size magnets will not be adequate. For instance, if we have to apply a magnet locally to an eye, we should naturally require a small size, preferably round magnet, which may cover the closed eye. A magnet of big size will neither be suitable nor advisable for application on the eye. On the other hand, if there is pain and swelling in a large portion of the body, in an area which is as big as the palm or still bigger, then the small magnet, which may be suitable for the eye, may not be sufficient for this painful area. A bigger-size magnet which can cover the painful and swollen area as far as possible, will be definitely better. Hence using the same magnet, with the same shape, size and design for application on different parts of body for relieving different types of diseases will neither be convenient nor suitable.

The same is the position about the strength of magnets. There are some tender places in our body, namely, brain, eye and heart where very powerful magnets should not be applied nor magnets of medium power should be kept in contact for long durations. On the other hand, low-power magnets may not be sufficient for the ailments of hard, large muscles or bones namely hips, thighs, knees or heels, etc. Thus the shape, size design and strength of a magnet should be selected according to the chronicity and seriousness of the disease, the part of the body affected and the age and the strength of the patient to bear the force of the magnetic emanations, when giving local treatment. It is better to keep these points in view while giving general treatment too.

It may be pointed out here that it is the magnetic force that relieves and cures diseases and not the dimensions of the magnet to be applied. Hence all magnets, prepared for commercial industrial, medical and other purposes can be utilised for the purpose of treatment, if their shapes, sizes, designs and strength are suitable for application to the part of the body affected and for the ailment of the case in hand.

The direction to which a magnetic pole faces, has bearing on the pattern of lines of force emanating from it. When North pole faces north, parallel lines of force emanate from it, while very few lines of force, in a distorted pattern, emanate if the North pole faces south or east or west. Similar is the position with the South pole.

Seating of Patients

It has been stated under the heading "Earth's magnetic effect on human beings", in Chapter 3, that over bodies are considered to have magnetic sides. In view of the position described therein, the seating of the patients when giving magnetic treatment, becomes important. The patients should be asked to sit in such a way that the North pole of the magnet when placed on the body, say on the forehead or throat, should be towards the North and the South pole of the magnet should be towards the South, if only one pole of a magnet is applied at a time. If the treatment is given by different poles of two magnets simultaneously, then the patient should be asked to sit facing 'West' so that his right hand and the whole right side remain towards the north and his left hand and the whole left side remain towards the south. If the patient is seated in these directions, the same magnets will show better results, than when the patient sits in other directions. In the suggested directions, the magnetic treatment will have the support of natural terrestrial magnetism also.

Peculiar Manifestations

Long experience with magnetic treatment shows that application of strong magnets causes some peculiar manifestations in some patients. Some people feel some mild tingling sensations as if some breeze is blowing or as if some light waves are passing in the hands or feet when strong magnets are applied to them. Some persons feel warmth, some feel giddiness, some get yawning, some feel sleepy and some get slight perspiration on the parts touching the magnets, while others do not feel any sensation. It is difficult to give any convincing explanation for the various feelings and manifestations, but the fact remains that whether one feels any sensation or not, the magnets work on every person touching them.

Duration of Application of Magnets

The magnetic treatment should normally be given for about
10 minutes only once a day. In chronic cases of Gout, Paralysis, Poliomyelitis, Rheumatism or Rheumatoid Arthritis, etc.,
the time of treatment can be gradually increased even up to
half-an-hour daily or for 15-20 minutes twice a day. In the
case of children, however, the time may be reduced upto
5 minutes a day, depending upon their age, disease and tenderness and the power of magnets.

There is no fixed course or time-limit for carrying out
magnetic treatment. It should be continued till cure is effected
The cure is achieved in different periods in different cases,
depending upon the nature and length of the disease, the age
and strength of the patient and the power of magnets to be
applied. In some cases, effect is noticed within a few days, in
some cases in about two weeks, in some chronic cases in a few
months. Magneic treatments corrects all functional disorders,
but in some very old and chronic cases, which have defied all
other treatments and where diseases of long standing have
caused considerable changes in the body, magnetic treatment
may also show little benefit, especially where organic changes
have set in. Some such cases may require surgery and some
others divine help.

Generally, there is no aggravation by magnetic treatment.
If, however, any pain seems to increase in the first instance in
any case, it may be due to the fact that the magnet in the
process of eliminating the pain, draws it out from the internal
parts of the body to the skin. The increase in pain, if felt in
any case, subsides in a short time and no separate treatment is
considered necessary for reducing it.

Different Ways of Application of Magnet

Dr. A.K. Bhattacharya of Naihati, West Bengal, has written
in his work on 'Magnet Healing' that when a powerful (Horse-
shoe) magnet is held in the left hand, it simultates the heart,
while in the right hand, the heart's action is slowed down. He
has demostrated the case of a patient to prove the correctness

of his theory. He adds that when there is high blood pressure, it means that the heart's action should be slowed down and hence the magnet should be held in the right hand and when the blood pressure is low, the magnet should be held in the left hand in order to increase the activity of the heart.

Dr. H.T. Bolakani has designed his patent magnet to be worn on the wrist of the left hand in all cases of all diseases. He prefers the left wrist as it is nearer the heart as compared with the right wrist. He has written in his book that many cases of high blood pressure have been relieved or cured by placing his magnet on the left wrist in all cases.

Dr. R. S. Thacker of Delhi advises that the treatment of high blood pressure should be carried out by Method I, namely, by applying magnets under both hands, but care should be taken to see that strong magnets are not applied to such persons for long periods. Treatment for five minutes in such cases may be sufficient. He feels that the magnet increases heat in the body. In high blood pressure, there is already heat and rush of blood to head. He, therefore, advises that a wet towel folded into several layers should be put on the lower part of the spine and it will quickly afford relief to the patient, if the blood pressure is very high, as that portion of the spine is directly connected with the head. In the case of low blood pressure, he places two magnets in the hands of the patients for 10 minutes or even longer and also applies South pole of a strong magnet on the lower part of the spine of such patients. Dr. Thacker's method of applying three magnets at a time corresponds to the method adopted by Dr. Mesmer in the treatment of a lady mentioned in Chapter 5, although for a different disease. Dr. Thacker sometimes applies even more than three magnets to a patient at the same time, if necessary.

The Aimante Trading Company of Tokyo, Japan, has made magnetic health band which is stated to be very useful against stiffness of shoulders and high blood pressure. They advise that the band should be worn on any of the arms, throughout the day and night. The magnetic band contains six to eight small ceramic magnets and looks like a watch strap or a bangle.

In view of the successes achieved by all the above magneto-therapists by applying magnets of different strengths to different parts of body for the same complaints, it can be assumed that the force of magnetism works on the body as a whole irrespective of the place on which it is applied. Thus it has remote effect also.

Guidelines and Precautions for Use of Magnets

(*i*) The best time for taking magnetic treatment is morning, after discharging usual routine duties and taking bath but before taking breakfast. If it is not possible to take this treatment in the morning for any reason, it may be taken in the evening before meals.

(*ii*) No cold thing should be drunk or eaten for at least half-an-hour after applying magnets. The magnets create temporary warmth in the body and it is not advisable to take anything cold when body is heated. Warm or hot things, namely milk or tea, etc. can, however, be taken immediately after application.

(*iii*) Bath should not be taken for 2 hours after application of strong magnets, for the same reason. Hence it is better to take magnetic treatment in the morning after taking bath.

(*iv*) Strong magnets should not be applied immediately after taking full meals as their application might induce nausea or vomiting in some cases.

(*v*) Strong magnets should not be applied to pregnant ladies, children and to delicate points in the body namely—brain, eyes, heart, etc.

(*vi*) Ordinarily, application of magnets does not show any harmful effects. But the application of strong magnets for a long time may result in some inconvenience, namely, heaviness in head, headache, sleepiness, yawning, tingling in nerves, etc. If any such inconvenience is felt, the contact of magnets should be discontinued immediately and the patient advised to take rest.

(*vii*) When the magnet has been improperly selected, the resulting sufferings can be permanently removed by lay-

laying the outspread hands on a large zinc plate for half-an-hour.

(*viii*) Homoeopathic medicine "Zincum Metallicum" antidotes the effects of the medicines prepared from the magnet. Hence this medicine can also be used, in low potencies, to antidote the adverse effect of application of magnets, noticed if any.

(*ix*) Opposite poles of strong flat magnets should not be clapped together. If they are placed face to face at all. fingers should not be allowed to come between them as they may be crushed.

(*x*) The opposite poles of two magnets may be joined together with a 'keeper' when they are not in use, so that their magnetism is not lost.

(*xi*) It is neither necessary nor advisable to remove gold and other ornaments from hands or fingers when using the magnets in palms.

(*xii*) The magnets should not however be allowed to come in contact with watches unless they are 'magnetic proof'.

TECHNIQUES OF APPLICATION OF MAGNETS IN THE TREATMENT OF 150 COMMON DISEASES

Sl. No.	Disease	Method to be applied	Remarks (M.W. stands for magnetised water)
1	2	3	4
1.	Abscess, Boils Cancers Carbuncles	I or V	Method I if disease is in upper part of the body ; method V if in lower part. Local treatment, with North Pole, should also be carried out on the spot of eruption.
2.	Acne	I	Local treatment with North Pole and drinking of M.W. will also help.
3.	Adenoids Nasal Polypus	I	-do-

1	2	3	4
4.	Anaemia	I	M.W. should be given to regulate and strengthen the normal function of the liver.
5.	Aphthae Thrush Ulcers in mouth	I	M.W. will also help as the ailment is generally due to disorders of stomach.
6.	Appendicitis (Not very acute)	—	Local treatment with South Pole of a strong magnet, twice daily.
7.	Appetite wanting	I	M.W. should also be given.
8.	Arthritis	I & V	Alternately on alternate days or morning and evening. Time may be increased gradually to 30 minutes in each sitting. M.W. will also help. Treatment should be continued for a long time.
9.	Asthma	I	Middle or High Power magnets for 10 minutes. M.W. to be given daily. Treatment for a long time as per details :

(*i*) A Pair of High Power magnets should be applied under palms for 10-12 minutes in the morning and for the same duration in the evening, if possible. (North pole under right palm & South pole under left palm). Continuous contact is necessary, without any pressure. This regulates circulatory, nervous and respiratory systems, proves beneficial in asthma and bronchitis, removes pain in chest and difficulty in breathing. If high power magnets are not available, medium power or premier magnets may be used but they are less powerful and should, therefore, be applied for 15 to 20 minutes.

(*ii*) The application of Crescent type (curved) Ceramic magnets is beneficial for the troubles of nose and throat. The north pole of these magnets should be applied on the right nostril, covering the full nasal wall, for about 10 minutes twice daily. This will gradually remove the problems of nose-namely blocking, polypus, sneezing, watering, etc. and will ease the difficulty in breathing through nose.

(*iii*) The crescent type ceramic magnets may also be applied on throat, for about 10 minutes once or twice daily. This will reduce coughing, irritation, pain and other inconveniences of throat, if any.

(*iv*) A Magnetic necklace may be worn around the neck touching the upper part of the chest. It has proved quite effective in asthma and bronchitis. The necklace can be worn throughout the day, except when taking bath. If some one does not like to wear it during the day, one may wear it during the night.

(*v*) The magnetised water prepared with High Power magnets should be drunk three/four times every day, about two ounces in each dose. The magnetised water not only removes congestion in chest and lungs, constipation and gasformation but also helps to regulate and improve appetite and digestion.

The above treatment can be combined with any medicine or exercise, etc. The treatment suggested above is primarily meant for bronchial asthma but is beneficial for allergic, cardiac and dry asthma also.

1	2	3	4
10.	Backache	Special	If horizontal, North pole on the right side and South pole on the left side ; if vertical, North pole on the upper portion .and South pole on the lower portion.
11.	Biliousness	Special	North pole below the liver and South pole opposite to it on the back. Method No. I will also help. M.W. is necessary.
12.	Biting of bees, Insects, scorpions,etc.	-do-	North pole on the affected part.
13.	Bladder affections	-do-	North pole on right side and South pole on left side of the abdomen, upon the bladder.
14.	Blood Pressure (High or Low)	I	In high blood pressure, treatment may be given for five minutes. Wet-cloth pad may be applied to the lowest part of the spinal cord if BP goes very high. In low blood pressure, treatment may be given for 15-20 minutes and one strong magnet may also be applied to the lower part of the spinal cord and M.W. may be given several times daily.
15.	Bronchitis (Brancho-pneumonia)	I	Treatment to be started with 5 minutes daily and time to be increased gradually up to

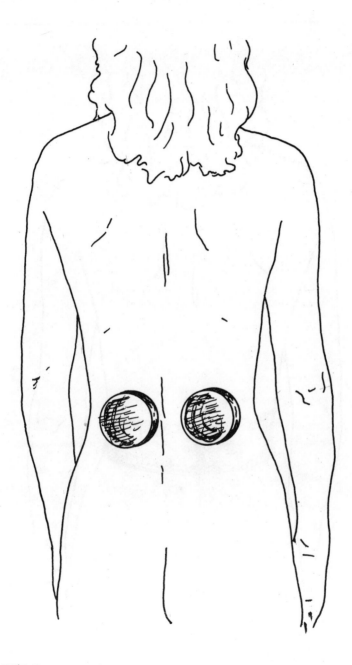

High Power Magnets on Back: For backache, lumbago, slipped disc & sprain etc. Apply the High Power Magnets on affected portion of the back.

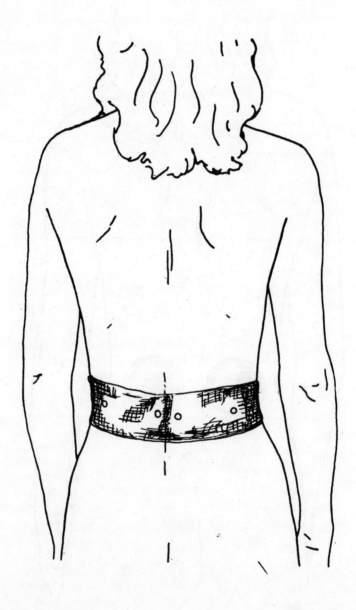

Back Belt: For backache, lumbago, pain, sprain, slipped disc, etc. Magnets should remain touching the affected part of the body.

1	2	3	4
			10 minutes. M.W. should be given. See Instructions for Asthma also.
16.	Cataract & Glaucoma	Special	Ceramic crescent-type magnets may be applied on both the eyes. If this does not help, treatment given at item No. 35 may be tried. These diseases can be benefitted in their initial stages only.
17.	Chilblains	I or V	If in hands, method I; if in feet, method V. If in all extremities, then methods I and V alternately, on alternate days, or in morning and evening.
18.	Cold in head	I	M.W. may be given every two hours. Cold things should be avoided.
19.	Colic	I	Local treatment with South pole also. M.W. too will help.
20.	Colitis	Local	High-powered magnets may be applied on the point of trouble and M.W. should be given.
21.	Constipation	II	The diagonal magnetic effect removes constipation in due course of time. M.W. must be given several times a day.

1	2	3	4
22.	Cough (dry or wet)	I	Small magnets may also be applied locally on the throat.
23.	Convulsions and Cramps	I or V	Remarks as against item 17.
24.	Corns in feet	V	M.W. of North pole will help.
25.	Coryza	I	Local treatment on nose also. M.W.
26.	Cuts	I & V	Local treatment also with North pole on the affected part.
27.	Dandruff	I	North pole of small magnets may also be applied on the head.
28.	Diabetes	I	If no benefit is felt in a few months, North pole on the pancreas and South pole behind it on the back. M.W. will help. Treatment to be continued for a long time.
29.	Diarrhoea and Dysentery	I	M.W. every two hours. Local treatment also if pain is there.
30.	Dropsy	I or V	Method I, if disease is more in upper part of the body ; method V, if disease is more in the lower part. M.W. will also help.
31.	Dyspepsia	I	Local treatment also. M.W. should be given, several times a day.

1	2	3	4
32.	Ear troubles (Boils in ears, deafness, discharge, Earache, Inflammation) ·	Special Treatment	South pole of a strong magnet may be applied under the right palm for 10 minutes and North pole of a medium or low-strength magnet near the affected ear. If trouble affects both ears, the small magnet may be applied near each ear for 5 minutes.
33.	Eczema, Herpes	I or V	Remarks as against Abscess. If weeping, a kerchief may be kept in the spot and magnet applied on the kerchief.
34.	Epilepsy, Fits	I	North pole to abdomen and South pole to back also. M.W. should be given several times a day and treatment should be continued for a long time.
35.	Eye troubles (all functional disorders)	Special Treatment*	South pole of a strong magnet may be applied under the right palm for 10 minutes and North pole of a low-strength magnet on each eye for 5 minutes irrespective of the nature ı of the disease. Treatment is the same for affections like conjunctivitis, defective vision, eye-lids inflammations, injuries to eye balls, iritis,

---

* **Note.** This is in accordance with the electric treatment of eyes given in the American Journal Service suggestions—Volume XXX No. 5 Sept., October, 1930.

1	2	3	4
			lachrymation, purulent discharge, short-or long-sightedness, sore eyes, spots before eyes, squint, etc.
36.	Facial paralysis	Special	Strong or Medium-powered magnets may be applied on the affected side of the face twice daily for 15 minutes each time and M.W. should be given.
37.	Falling and greying of hair	I	Low-powered magnets should also be applied on both the temples. M.W. given to drink and use of soaps should be avoided.
38.	Fevers	I	Medium-powered magnets should be applied in the morning and evening for 5 minutes and M.W. should be given to drink every two hours.
39.	Fistula	V	North pole of a small magnet may also be applied or tied to the point of fistula if possible. M.W. should be given.
40.	Fissures	V	Small magnets may also be used or tied on the fissures at night.
41.	Flatulence (gas, wind)	I	Medium-powered magnets may also be applied on the abdomen if there is pain. M.W. is a must for such cases. Ginger

1	2	3	4
			(*Adrak*) should be given in plenty and gas producing things avoided.
42.	Foreign material in body	Local	If pins or needless, etc. get into the body, strong magnets should be applied immediately to the point of pricking so that the pins, etc., may be attracted and taken out by the magnets. If they go deep into the body, there is no alternative but to get the portion X-Rayed and operated.
43.	Gall stones	I	North pole on liver region M.W. must be given to drink several times a day. Local treatment for pain, if any.
44.	Giddiness	I	M.W. will be an additional help.
45.	Goitre	I	Medium-powered or crescent-type magnets should also be applied locally on the swollen thyroid gland. Bananas and M.W. should be taken by the potient. Treatment should continue for a long time.
46.	Gout	I & V	Method I or V according to location, or alternately on alternate days or in the morning and evening. Treatment may be given twice daily and should be continued for a long time. M.W. necessary.

1	2	3	4
47.	Gravel (deposits in urine/red or white)	V	M.W. several times a day, for a long time as it helps to wash out deposits and stones from bladder, and kidneys. Local treatment also if pain is there.
48.	Gums— bleeding and receding	Special	Low-powered magnets may be applied on the affected teeth, outside the mouth.
49.	Headache (different types)	According to causes	(*i*) If due to indigestion, method I, and M.W.

(*ii*) If due to toxaemia : (A) Jaundice, method I ; (B) Nephritis, method V (C) Sinusitis, ceramic-magnets on nose ; (D) Tonsilitis, magnets on throat, etc.,

(*iii*) If due to fevers, method I and M.W. every two hours,

(*iv*) If due to ear trouble, treatment as for ear trouble,

(*v*) If due to eye trouble, treatment as for eye troubles,

(*vi*) If due to mental strain, or worry, Method I for 15-20 minutes, & M.W.

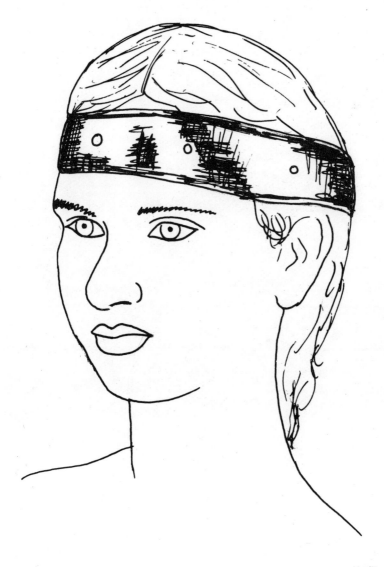

Magnetic Head-Belt: On Forehead for headache, hemicrania, migraine and insomnia. Apply the belt covering both the temples and the Forehead.

1	2	3	4
			(*vii*) If due to injury, local treatment on injured portion, and
			(*viii*) If cause not known, crescent-type magnets on forehead. North pole on right-side and South pole on left-side and Magnetised water.
50.	Heart trouble (Angina, Palpitation, Sinking, weakness)	I	A small magnet may also be applied near the troubled area for 5 minutes only and its effect may be watched. Strong magnets should *not* be applied on the heart and head.
51.	Hepatitis	I	Local treatment with South pole also along with M.W.
52.	Hernia	I	Local treatment with South pole is necessary. M.W. also.
53.	Hiccough	I	Another method is to apply the North pole of a strong magnet on the abdomen and South pole, just opposite to it, on the back. M.W. also.
54.	Hoarseness	I	Crescent-type magnets also on throat and M.W. several times.
55.	Hydrocele	V	M.W. is essential. Local treatment with South pole is also advisable.

1	2	3	4
56.	Hyperacidity	I & II	Local treatment with both poles and M.W. are also advisable.
57.	Hypochondria	I	M.W. several times a day.
58.	Hysteria	II	North pole above the uterus and South pole below it. M.W. also.
59.	Increasing height	Special	North pole of crescent-type magnet on forehead and South pole on back of head. Next day, North pole may be shifted to above the right ear and South pole above the left ear. This will give strength to the Pituitary gland which controls the height. Long treatment.
60.	Influenza	I	Remarks as against Fevers.
61.	Injuries	I or V	According to location ; but local treatment is more useful and should be given immediately. Hot things and M W. should be given to eat and drink and cold things should be avoided.
62.	Insomnia	V (In Evening)	One small magnet, preferably South pole, on Centre of forehead at bed time also.
63.	Intelligence (to increase)	I	One small magnet, preferably South pole of crescent type on forehead also.

1	2	3	4
64.	Jaundice	I	M.W. must be given. Local treatment with small or MP magnets is advisable. Papaya, radish and cane juice are beneficial in this disease.
65.	Kidney Pain (renal colic)	I	Local treatment is a MUST. M.W. will help and should be given for free urination.
66.	Leucoderma	I or V	According to location of disease. If only one or two patches, local treatment with South pole.
67.	Liver enlargement	I	Small South pole magnet on spot and M.W. also.
68.	Locomotor ataxia	Special	North pole on the upper part and South pole on the lower part of the spinal cord.
69.	Lumbago	V	One strong magnet (South pole) may be applied on the painful spot also.
70.	Lymphatic glands (swelling of)	I and V	Local treatment on swollen glands also. M.W.
71.	Malaria	I	Remarks as against fevers.
72.	Measles	I	Treatment as for fevers.
73.	Memory (weak)	I	Treatment as for increasing Intelligence.

1	2	3	4
74.	Mental retardation	I	Treatment as for increasing Intelligence.
75.	Meningitis	I	Local treatment on both sides of neck also.
76.	Migraine	I	Low-powered magnets over the eyebrows or on temples also.
77.	Mumps	I	Local treatment with crescent-type magnets also, morning and evening, for a few days.
78.	Nephritis	V	Local treatment over kidneys also. M.W., frequent doses of it is a MUST in this disease.
79.	Neuralgia, Neurasthenia, Neuritis	I	Local treatment with South pole also where possible. M.W. will help.
80.	Obesity	I & V	Four strong magnets may be applied simultaneously and their effect may be watched or two magnets may be applied first under palms (I) and then under soles method (V). Diet should be restricted, fats may be avoided and M.W. should be given.
81.	Orchitis	I	Local treatment with South pole is beneficial.
82.	Osteo-arthritis	I & V	Local treatment with strong magnets is also necessary for a long time.

1	2	3	4
83.	Palpitation	I	Remarks as against Heart trouble. M.W. will help.
84.	Paralysis	I & V	Alternately on alternate days. If only on right side of whole body, method No. IV ; and if only on left side of whole body, method No. III. Time may be increased gradually up to 30 minutes or treatment may be given twice daily upto 15 minutes each time. Treatment should be continued for a long time. M.W. should be given regularly.
85.	Piles (Haemorrhoids)	V	M.W. may be given continuously. Patient may also sit over a pair of strong magnets.
86.	Pleurisy	I	M.W. may be given continuously, for a long period.
87.	Pneumonia	I	Treatment as for Fevers. Small magnets may also be applied on painful parts if any.
88.	Poliomyelitis	V	Local treatment should also be given. N.P. on hip, S.P. under sole. See remarks against Paralysis.
89.	Pox (Chicken on Small)	I	Treatment same for both. M.W. every two hours.
90.	Prostate enlargement	V	Local treatment for a long time, with South pole, M.W. should also be given regularly.

1	2	3	4
91.	Pyorrhea	I	See item 48 also.
92.	Rheumatism	I & V	Also see remarks against Paralysis. Treatment for a long time.
93.	Ringworm		Treatment as per item Nos. 1 and 33.
94.	Sciatica	V	Local treatment on painful portion. Alternatively, apply North pole on the affected hip and South pole under the relevant foot.
95.	Sexual Weakness (Males)	V	Also apply North pole below the navel and South pole below it, above the male organ. Patient may also sit over the magnets keeping them side by side.
96.	Sinusitis	Local	Apply crescent-type magnets on both sides of nose or on the painful place.
97.	Slipped disc	Special	North pole on the upper part of the spinal cord where the pain starts and South pole on the spot of the severe pain on lumber region, or N.P. on right side of back and S.P. on left side of back.
98.	Sneezing	-do-	As for sinusitis.
99.	Spermatorrhea		As per item No. 95 above.

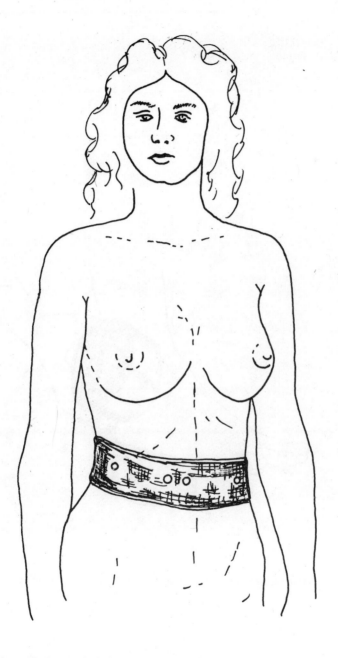

Magnetic Stomach-Belt for abdominal ailments, for pain, swelling, hernia, and backache, etc.

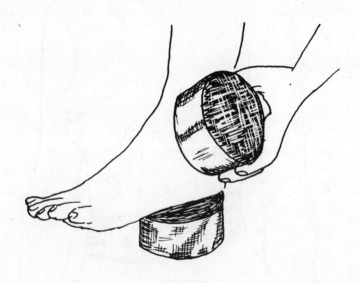

For Swollen, Stiff and Painful Ankle: North Pole on the affected ankle and South Pole under the heel.

1	2	3	4
100.	Spleen enlargement	I	Local treatment with South pole. M.W. will also help.
101.	Stiffness of neck	Special	North pole on the back of the neck and South pole on the other end of the stiffness.
102.	Stomach trouble (all diseases)	II	The diagonal effect of magnetism relieves all troubles of liver, stomach, spleen, abdomen, intestines, etc. M.W. must be given with it, for a long time.
103.	Stones	I & V	If in the gall-bladder, method No. I, if in the kidney, method No. V. M.W. must be given with it. N.P. on painful part.
104.	Swelling of legs & feet	V	M.W. is a MUST and should continue for a long time. Use of salt should be minimised.
105.	Syphilis and Gonorrhea	V	M.W. mixed with equal quantity of simple water may also help in both diseases. Treatment should continue for a long time.
106.	Tonsilitis, Pharyngitis	I	Local treatment on throat also. Crescent-type magnets may be used. Cold and sour things should be avoided.
107.	Tuberculosis	I	M.W. is essential.
108.	Typhoid	I	Remarks as against fevers.

1	2	3	4
109.	Ulcers in Abdomen Peptic, Gastric or duodinal	I	M.W. may be given every two hours. Chillies should be avoided. Local application will also help.
110.	Urethritis	V	Magnets may be applied on urethra also. M.W. must be given.
111.	Urinary diseases	V	For scanty or stoppage of urine, give one ounce of magnetised water, with one ounce of simple water in quick succession of say 5 minutes for an hour or two and the patient will pass urine.
112.	Urticaria	I & V	Medium or strong magnets should be used. M.W. will also help.
113.	Veins (inflammed, varicose)	I or V	According to location of disease. Local treatment also.
114.	Vomiting	I	M.W. every half an hour or so.
115.	Worms	II	M.W. should be given to drink 3-4 times every day.
116.	Wounds	Local	After dressing, magnets may be applied on wounds for quick healing. South pole.
117.	Wry neck	Special	Magnets to be applied locally on the bent neck.

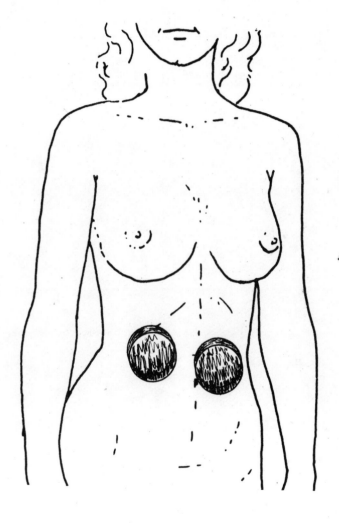

Ovaries: For Pain, Swelling, Stiffness, Dysmenorrhea and other female disorders including leucorrhea.

DISEASES OF WOMEN

1	2	3	4
118.	Amenorrhoea (late/scanty menses)	V	M.W. should also be given. Treatment should continue for a long time.
119.	Bearing down (falling of womb)	V	South pole may also be applied below the navel. M.W. should be given three-four times daily,
120.	Breast-tumour	Local	South pole may be applied on the tumour, if no infection.
121.	Cysts or inflammation	I or V	Local treatment also, along with M.W.
122.	Dysmenorrhoea (painful menses)	V	Magnets may also be applied on abdomen and M.W. should be given.
123.	Hysteria	V	North pole above the uterus and South pole below it, if disorder in menses is also there.
124.	Inflammation of womb or ovaries	V	Local treatment also. M.W. should be given regularly.
125.	Labour pains (or after pains)	I	Local treatment will also be beneficial. M.W. should be given.
126.	Leucorrhoea	I & V	Alternately on alternate days. M.W. will also help.
127.	Loss of sexual desire.	Special	Treatment as per item 123.

1	2	3	4
128.	Mastitis	I	South pole on the affected nipple.
129.	Menopause (troubles of)	V	Remarks as against Amenorrhoea.
130.	Ovarian cyst or tumour	Local	North pole on right side and South pole on left side of abdomen.
131.	Prolapsus uteri	V	South pole below the uterus.
132.	Pruritis vulvae	V	Magnets may be applied on both the external sides of uterus.
133.	Sore nipples	I	Small magnets may be applied on nipples also.

DISEASES OF CHILDREN

1	2	3	4
134.	Atrophy (Wasting)	I & V	Alternately. M.W. should be given to improve general health.
135.	Bed wetting	V	-do-
136.	Cholera, Diarrhoea	I	M.W. every half an hour or so.
137.	Crusta lactea	I	Small magnets may be applied on head also.
138.	Dentition troubles	I	Remarks as against item 134.
139.	Itching in nose	Special	Ceramic magnets may be applied on both sides of nose.

1	2	3	4
140.	Milk curds in stools/vomits	I	Remarks as against item 136.
141.	Night terrors	I	Remarks as against item 134.
142.	Prolapsus ani	V	The child may be asked to sit on the pair of M.P. magnets.
143.	Rickets	I	M.W. may also be given 3-4 times.
144.	Snuffles	Special	Treatment as per item No. 139.
145.	Stoppage of nose	I	-do-
146.	Strabismus (Squint)	Special	Two small crescent-type magnets may be applied on both the eyes. North pole on the right eye and South pole on the left eye. If this does not work satisfactorily, then the method suggested at item 35 may be adopted.
147.	Umbilicus, bleeding or inflammation	I	If bleeding then North pole, if inflammation then South pole on the umbilicus.
148.	Vomiting	I	M.W. half-an-hourly or one hourly.
149.	Whooping cough	I	Ceramic magnets may be applied below the throat twice or thrice or even more times everyday.
150.	Wind in stomach	I	Ceramic magnets may also be applied on abdomen and M.W. should be given.

The cases of diseases not mentioned here may be treated on the basis of general guidelines and according to the location of the ailments.

Similarly, the diseases of women and children not detailed under these headings may be dealt with according to the suggestions given in the list of general diseases.

The application of magnets does not show the same improvement in all cases of the same disease. The response differs according to length and seriousness of the disease and the age and strength of the patient.

Almost all diseases can be cured, or at least relieved, by magnetotherapy, provided any organic defects have not set in. The improvement does not, however show a steady course in chronic ailments and there may be ups and downs for various reasons, but the degree of improvement and its duration increases till it becomes a lasting cure.

It may be reiterated here that the guidelines and the precautions suggested in this chapter should be observed before and after application of strong magnets, in all cases, as far as possible.

The rules and methods given above are only general rules. There may be exceptions also in exceptional cases. Hence, the Magnetotherapists treating the cases may exercise their own intelligence on the basis of general instructions given herein and take their own decision to apply magnets of suitable strength in any particular case as they consider suitable.

11

Magnetised Water

Characteristics of Water

Water is a transparent fluid, which has no colour, odour, shape or taste of its own. It takes the shape of its container and the colour, odour and taste of other things mixed with it. Thus it has got the characteristic of assimilating the properties of other things. Accordingly, when the properties of a magnet are absorbed in water by continuous contact between the two, the water gets magnetised and shows its beneficial effect in almost all ailments when taken internally for some considerable time.

Influence of Magnetic Field on Properties of Water

Scientists have proved that a magnetic field influences the progress of crystallisation in solutions and increases the number of crystallisation centres. It has also been established that many physical and chemical properties of water undergo a change when it is exposed even for fractions of a second to the influence of a weak magnetic field. The changes take place in its boiling temperature, density, electrical conductivity, surface tension and viscosity and the new properties exist for several days.

Useful Results of Experiments with Magnetised Water

Many experiments have been made in Russia with magnetised water and very useful results have been noticed in different fields of technology. A brief description of some industries where magnetised water has been found particularly beneficial is given below :

It is a matter of common knowledge that when water flows into a pipeline, some deposits adhere to the walls of the pipes.

These deposited coatings of the pipes and other fittings cause a great nuisance, interfere with the free working of the machinery and reduce its efficiency. These deposits are harmful for combustion engines also. A coating of 1.5 mm in thickness reduces the power of a car engine by 5 horse power. Consequently, the expenditure of fuel and lubricants is increased and the mechanical strength of various parts of the engine is decreased.

When a section of a pipeline carrying water is placed in a magnetic field, there appears on its walls, a brownish powder instead of the coating of hard deposit. This powder can be removed from the pipes, fittings, or the boilers, etc. without stopping the technological process.

Magnetised water has helped the automobile engineers. When poured into radiators, it prevents the forming of deposits and also destroys old salt sediments on the pipes. The magnetised water also removes the so-called water stone inside the pipes and fittings.

Magnetised water has proved useful for oil industry. Salts adhere to the pipes through which oil is pumped out to the surface. Sets of magnets were mounted in the shafts of walls. This resulted in the dropping of the sedimentation of salts in pipes and in the manifold increase of their length of service.

Magnetised water lessens dust during the drilling of blast holes and thus improves the working condition of the miners.

Magnetised water helps in building construction too. The strength of samples of concrete made with magnetised water is increased by about 20 to 35 per cent. Light concretes become almost twice stronger and heavy concretes 50 per cent stronger as compared to similar concretes made with ordinary water. Naturally, magnetised water reduces the expenditure on concretes.

Magnetised water was also used in irrigation and the plants grew at a speed 20 to 40 per cent faster than before.

The magnetic treatment of water thus saves a lot of expenses of labour, time and money and is successfully applied in many industries in Russia.

It appears that the use of magnetised water can solve or minimise many problems and can afford many facilities. The use of magnetised water, therefore, deserves the attention of the industrialists in India for the benefit of their industries and for the country as a whole.

Beneficial Effects of Magnetised Water on Human Beings

Let us now come to the beneficial use of magnetised water in the diseases of human beings.

The live tissues are mostly colloidal solutions. Scientists have, therefore, arrived at the conclusion that the magnetic field can influence biological processes as well.

It has been shown in previous chapters that the force of magnetism has a great influence on the living organisms. If the invisible force of magnetism is transferred to some other substance which is capable of absorbing it within itself, and then the magnetised substance is administered into and in assimilated by any living organism, such assimilation naturally has its effect on the living organism.

When a permanent magnet is kept in continuous contact with water, for considerable time, the water is not only influenced by the magnetic flux of the magnet, but becomes magnetised and acquires magnetic properties. Such magnetised water has its effect on the human body when taken internally, regularly for a considerable period.

Magnetised Water helps in All Diseases

The experience on long use of magnetised water, prepared from the healing vibrations of permanent magnets, has proved beyond doubt that it helps in almost all diseases and is especially beneficial in the disorders of the digestive, nervous and urinary systems.

The continuous use of magnetised water improves digestion, increases appetite and reduces excess of acids and bile. It helps in proper movement of bowels and expels poison, unwarranted salts and morbidity from the body.

The use of magnetised water has helped women in the regularisation of their menses.

The magnetised water can also help to clear the clogged arteries, normalise circulatory system and regulate the functioning of the heart.

The magnetised water helps in kidney troubles and brings out urine. If urine is stopped, administration of one ounce of the magnetised water mixed with one ounce of simple water in quick succession of 5 to 10 minutes for 8 to 10 times will make the patient pass urine. In a Leningrad clinic, patients suffering from stones in the kidneys and gall bladder drank magnetised water and it helped to wash out the salts and stones from their organism.

The magnetised water is effective in the treatment of all kinds of fevers, all sorts of pains, asthma, bronchitis, colds, coughs, headaches, etc. In short, it helps in the removal of every indisposition.

The use of magnetised water is economical, safe and simple. Magnetised water can be easily prepared in every house if some magnets are available. Magnetised water can be taken by healthy persons also for improving digestion and for removing weakness and tiredness associated with the day-to-day activity of life.

Dr. H.T. Bolakani has written in his book "Secrets of Magnet Therapy" that many Europeans go to a place "Evian" in France to seek relief from various ailments of the kidneys, exhaustion, gout and obesity, as well as prematurely growing old. Every cure is based there on Evian Water, which flows from a spring. Bottles of this water are sold all over France and it shares honours in houses and restaurants with other mineral waters. This water is proclaimed beneficial for feeding children, diuresis, disintoxication, kidney troubles, arthiritis, gout, obesity and urinary ailments. It is felt that Evian Water is nothing else but 'Magnetised Water'.

It has been reported that patients in Britain, Denmark, Norway and Sweden have noticed that drinking magnetised water or even Beer treated with magnetic conditioner has improved their health. The Russians call the magnetised water as 'Wonder Water'.

Milk can be Magnetised and Made more Potential

Many people in India are in the habit of taking milk before going to sleep at night. If a glass of hot milk is kept over the South Pole of a permanent magnet, encased in a round or square frame about 3 or 4 inches diameter, or if two permanent magnets of crescent type of about 5 cms. length are placed around and in close contact with the glass, for 20 to 30 minutes, and the milk is taken thereafter, it makes a very beneficial diet for the convalescent period and becomes more potential generally as well as sexually.

A news item about the effect of magnets and magnetised water has been published in the Times of India and the Hindustan Times both dated the 21st August 1975. The news is reproduced below for information :

New Delhi—August 20—Soviet researchers have found that cows give more milk when magnetised.

They have discovered that magnets can raise milk output and the fat content in milk, according to the Soviet News Agency—APN. They have reported that magnetic treatment also cures and prevents a disease called 'Mastitis'.

Magnetised water is also used to cure human ailments. It is used in Soviet Clinics to relieve pain, reduce swelling and for the removal and prevention of kidney stones.

"Some Soviet biologists are of the view that all effects of magnetism on living beings are exerted through water"—PTI.

Preparation of Magnetised Water

There are different views about the methods of preparation of magnetised water. Some of the methods are given below for information :

Some Magnetotherapists are of the view that an iron-alloy magnet of one piece, which can lift a quarter of a kilogram of iron-weight, may be taken and cleaned thoroughly. If the magnet has any colour paint, it should be removed completely. Then a glass-tumbler may be taken and filled up with clean drinking water. The magnet may be immersed in the water and the glass tumbler may be covered and kept safely. This may be done in the evening. The water gets magnetised in a short time. The magnet may, however, be allowed to remain in the water for twelve hours to assimilate full magnetic emanations. Next Morning the magnetised water may be filtered and transferred to a clean colourless bottle from which it may be used.

Some other magnetotherapists are of the view that if a bigger one-piece iron-alloy magnet which can lift about one kilogram of iron-weight, is used for preparation of magnetised water, bigger glass-vessel or china-clay jar which can contain 2 or 3 litres of water may be used. The method of preparation of magnetised water remains the same in both the ways. The magnetised water prepared in the bigger vessel or jar may be kept in several bottles after filteration and can be used by many persons or by one person for many days. The duration of keeping the magnet in the bigger vessel or jar also remains the same.

The magnet can also be allowed to remain in water for 24 hours, but during this time or any longer period, there is the likelihood of the magnet getting rusted and the water getting contaminated in both of these ways. It is, therefore, necessary that the magnet and the glass tumbler or the jar, in which the magnet is kept, must be cleaned thoroughly every time before keeping the magnet in water.

In case any reddish deposit is seen in the glass-tur..bler or in the jar or in the bottles, in which the magnetised water is stored after filteration, the magnetised water up to a centimetre above the bottom of the bottle may be used for human consumption and the lower reddish portion of the water may be

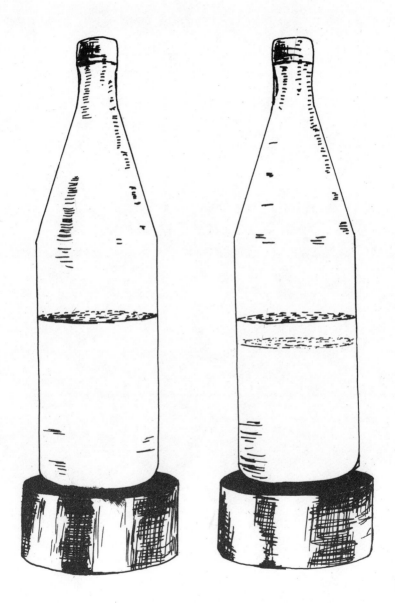

MAGNETISED WATER: Water is being Magnetised on both poles.
Useful for improving appetite and digestion, helps in reducing constipation
and gas formation, also brings out urine and washes out stone from Kidneys.

thrown or given to the roots of plants or trees. The glass jar or the bottle may be cleaned for further storage of fresh magnetised water. It is no use keeping the magnet in water for a longer period as it will only lead to contamination without any further advantage, because 24 hours are quite sufficient to fully magnetise the water.

In order to completely avoid the possibility of rusting of the magnet and contamination of the water, the magnet may be kept in close contact with the vessel (glass-tumbler or glass-jar from outside as suggested for magnetising milk.)

A magnet of the same or bigger size may be taken for this purpose. Magnetism passes through glass, and, therefore, milk, water, wine, juice, etc., assimilate magnetic effect even when magnets are kept in close touch with the vessels from outside. The glass-tumbler or the glass-jar may be kept either by the side of or over the magnet for at least 12 hours, or upto 24 hours without any risk of rust or contamination. For this purpose, magnets enclosed in flat, round or square metal covers of the diameter of 7.5 to 10 cms. are most suitable as the glass-tumblers or glass-jars can be easily kept over them and the magnetic emanations pass into the water through the full bottom of the containers.

My own practice has been to follow the method last mentioned *i.e.* to keep the magnets outside the container and not to put them in the water.

I take a pair of encased magnets of round flat surface with a diameter of 7 to 10 centimetres (3-4 inches) having different poles in their centres and two glass bottles or jars. I fill the bottles or jars with fresh drinking water and keep one bottle or jar on the centre of the one magnet and the other bottle or jar on the centre of the other magnet in the evening. The containers are properly covered. The water gets magnetised during the night. As a further step towards precaution or purity, the water is boiled and then cooled before filling the bottles or jars. Then the water of both the containers is transferred to a clean third container. The combined magnetised water is ready for use.

My method has no risk of rusting of magnets or contamination of the water.

The magnets used by me for magnetising water are the same magnets which I use for giving magnetic treatment under palms and soles, as these encased magnets have a diameter of 10 centimetres (about 4 inches). Full bottles or jars can be conveniently kept over them and the same magnets prove quite suitable for this purpose also. The magnetic emanations pass into the water through the full bottom of the containers and the water becomes fully magnetised.

Dosage of Magnetised Water

The dose of magnetised water for adults is two ounces (about 50 ml.) at a time. It may best be taken in the morning before breakfast and after both the major meals. For children, the dosage may be reduced to one ounce at a time, thrice daily, and in the case of infants it may be further reduced to one or two teaspoonfuls at a time, thrice daily.

In fever, a dose of the magnetised water be taken every two hours. It may, however, be noted that magnetised water, with magnetic properties becomes a medicine and should not be taken in excessive quantities like simple plain water.

Russian Way of Magnetising Water

It is understood that the Russians magnetise their water in a peculiar way. They hang a bottle of water up on a suitable stand and place a simple valve in the bottle end and adjust the valve to allow drops, not a stream of water, but drops of water to drop as drops, as fast as possible without its turning into a stream of water, placing then a horse-shoe magnet so that the drops of water will drop and pass through the ends of the two poles of this type of magnets. Then they collect the water in another bottle or jar below the magnets used. Then using the water, they soon discovered that the water gave an uplift in the physical senses of man.

Whatsoever the method may be followed in Russia for magnetising the water but it is seen that they pass the water through both the poles of the magnet. This is quite in keeping with magnetising the water with both the poles as done by me.

American Way of Magnetising Water

The Americans have confirmed the Russian opinion that the properties of water change when it is polarised or magnetised. They have also confirmed that the Russians have been using polarised water in their hospitals for years. The Americans, however, follow a different procedure for magnetising water. They pass water through the North Pole of the bar or cylindrical magnet and this water magnetised with the single pole only helped to heal the bed sores, if the sores were washed with this water everyday. This water added to heal the sore quicker and the sore remained healed up later also.

They later found that a far better and very simple way could be used to polarise water. They took the plastic jug with a capacity of one gallon with a tight cap, filled it up with plain tap water and placed it on the North Pole of a long bar or a cylindrical magnet of 1000 gauss against one side of the jug for 20 to 30 minutes. They got a fine gallon of magnetically treated water. They also found that leaving the magnet against the jug all the time day and night and adding water as they used it, was the most simple method and also most practical. After long experience of several years, they found that after using this water for a number of years, its value to them has been rewarding and outstanding in effects.

The Americans have announced their findings of what happens to the water when it is magnetised, as follows :

When the Americans turned to testing for the amounts of oxygen that water is chemically composed of, then they found an interesting discovery namely that the oxygen level was lower in the treated water than it was in untreated water. There was also a change in the hydrogen ion, electronic activity ; the hydrogen ions that is the charged articles were altered to a degree to present a noticeable higher state of activity. This fact was checked several times and many tests were done. But the results were the same.

The upgrading of the activity of the hydrogen in water was also seen and can be supported. Even greater discoveries have since been seen made in altering the hydrogen in oxygen activity of water. With the additional magnetic fields greater changes are noted.

It has also been noted that when water is treated with simple North or South Pole only we make it safer for human consumption, even if the water might be stale or cold or stored for any length of time.

Magnetic Treatment of Water in Japan

The Japanese scientists have pressed that the fluids change their weight when placed in magnetic fields. The reason for this reduction in weight is still not known and is being investigated.

Part V

12

Advantages of Magnetotherapy

Strong Medicines have Strong Reactions

It is well known that strong medicines of the modern age have their strong reactions and sometimes result in fatal consequences. It is only the systems of treatment based on natural laws and principles which do not show harmful side effects.

The practitioners of every system of medicine plead and emphasis that while a patient is under their care and is taking their medicines, no other treatment should be given to him side by side, but magnetotherapy does not follow the above general convention.

Magnetotherapy is Natural Treatment

This system of treatment is based on natural laws, works in conformity with the nature and is an aid to natural processes of healing. It has, therefore, no harmful effects which could endanger the life of a patient.

The treatment through magnets can be taken alone or along with any other treatment, as it does not interfere with any medical system but helps to accelerate the action of all medicines which have the effect of restoring the ailing body to its normal state in a natural way.

Magnetic Touch Accelerates Blood Circulation

The continuous contact with magnets for some time generates warmth in body, activates the whole working system and accelerates blood circulation. It, therefore, gives strength and tones up the body as a whole, helps in faster recovery from ailments, removes, tiredness, weakness, proves beneficial in convalescence periods and reduces pains and swellings of every part of the body.

Magnetic Treatment is Beneficial for Light Conditions as well as for Serious Diseases

The treatment with magnets helps those who are not mentally satisfied with their lives. It assists those who want more out of living, who live in quiet depression but feel that there is a better way of life. It is beneficial for the hurried, tense business executive, the worried nervous house wife, the career women unable to find mental peace, the child who is enraged by continued temper tantrums, the man and woman who cannot stop drinking or living of pills, and for the lonely and the hypochondriac. If such persons take advantage of magnetism, they will find it rewarding, changing their lives for the better.

But magnetotherapy is not only for the treatment of light conditions mentioned above. It has cured a large number of cases of serious sickness, which were considered incurable and were given up by efficient doctors. It has cured many of the so-called incurable diseases like cancer, chronic arthritis, eczema, high blood pressure, poliomyelitis, prostate enlargement, rheumatism, sleeplessness, etc., as stated briefly in the cases given in Chapters 14 and 15. Relieving severe toothache in one or two sittings with magnets for 10-15 minutes is a common feature of magnetotherapy.

Beneficial for All Ages and Both Sexes

The treatment, through the application of magnets, is so simple that it can be given or taken at any time, at any place and at any part of the body. It can be taken by every person without any consideration of age or sex.

Very Quick Relief in Some Cases

This treatment proves so effective and its effect is so quick and lasting that sometimes only one sitting with magnets is sufficient and a second sitting is not needed, as often happens in the case of recent pains—especially in toothache, sprains, etc.

No Preparations

One does not have to make any preparation to give or take this treatment as it is done only by touching the magnets for some time.

The treatment has to be taken only once a day—generally for 10 minutes.

The magnets can be kept at home and can be taken to the shop, factory or office where one may be working. The treatment can be taken during long journey too.

No water or tea or milk or anything else of the sort is required for this treatment as no medicine is to be taken internally under this system of treatment.

The same magnets can be used by so many patients, each day, without washing, cleaning or disinfecting them. The same magnets can be used for all complaints, if the size, shape, design and power of the magnets are suitable for the parts of the body where they are to be applied and for the diseases to be treated.

No Recurring Expenditure

Once a pair of magnets is obtained, there is no recurring expenditure. Hence this treatment saves a lot of expenditure on medical bills.

Saving of Time

It also saves one a lot of trouble and time otherwise spent in going to hospitals, dispensaries and to private doctors, standing there in long queues and waiting for hours.

The cures effected by magnetic treatment are long lasting as this system works by scientifically correcting the various natural systems functioning in the body.

No Habit Forming

This treatment is not habit forming. If the user of magnets does not use them for some days or weeks, he does feel anything wanting or any urge for using them.

Magnets Keep Their Users Fresh, Energetic and Youthful

The magnets keep their users, including ladies and children, fresh, energetic and youthful ; and these qualities go a long way to enable them to maintain and improve their health and to look handsome and beautiful all the year round.

A magnet may be applied to any part of the body and its effect will reach everywhere in the body through the circulatory and nervous systems ; of course it will be immediate and a little more at the part of the body where the magnet is applied.

Effectively draws Pain out of the Body

Every disease is associated with some kind of pain. A magnet has special property of alleviating and removing pain from any cause and helps the human organism to return to normalcy. Hence treatment with magnets has a wide field of action in all diseases and can correct all the functional disorders of the body by removing pain and providing soothing effect in every ailment. It is, therefore, specially beneficial in all diseases which cause any kind of pain in the body.

The treatment with magnets does not cause any shock or aggravation as is sometimes observed in some other systems of treatment.

The permanent magnets, which are the tools of the treatment, retain their power for a very long time, namely, for several years. If they lose their power in due course of time, they can be recharged to regain their lost magnetism. Thus the magnets never get too old so as to be discarded and thrown away as unserviceable at any time.

Precautionary and Prophylactic Use of Magnets

The treatment with magnets can be taken by healthy persons also, daily or occasionly, as a precautionary measure. They would feel tranquil and will not feel fatigued at the fag end of the day.

The treatment with magnets can be taken as a prophylactic measure against many infectious diseases like measles, chicken pox, influenza, etc. Magnetised water is an additional help in the treatment of every disease. If magnetised water is taken every four hours during an epidemic, it can save the user from contracting any such disease ; and in case the infection has already been caught, the duration and severity of the disease will be surprisingly reduced. Magnetised water can be easily prepared in every house, with a single pair of magnets only, as suggested in the previous chapter on 'Magnetised Water.'

Side-Effects

Dr. A.K. Bhattacharya of Naihati, West Bengal, has written in his book 'Magnet and Magnetic Field', on the basis of a report on Biomagnetism from the Delaware Laboratories Limited, Oxford, England, that there were no noticeable side-effects of the experiments carried out by them. They were, however, able to elicit the following few probable ones through careful questioning :

(*i*) Tiredness after initial treatment but not thereafter.

(*ii*) Diuresis immediately following treatment, but not sustained.

(*iii*) Healthier bowel action in those subjects who sometimes suffered from sluggishness.

(*iv*) More rapid healing of small cuts and abrasions and rapid reduction of inflammation.

(*v*) A beneficial effect in some young subjects with acne.

(*vi*) Some female subjects reported a loss of weight during magnetic treatment and a reduction in adipose tissue (fat cells) about the thighs.

It will be observed that only the first side-effect could be considered slightly harmful but that temporary effect was also felt only after the initial treatment, not thereafter. All the other side-effects were beneficial.

While considering the side effects, it may be reiterated that Dr. Maclean of New York noticed that one interesting side-effect of repeated exposure of magnetism on human being was the restoration of pigmentation in hair of many of his patients from a silvery white to its former natural colour.

Magnetic Treatment Beneficial for People of All Humours and Characteristics

The following statement of the great physican, Paracelsus, regarding the therapeutic uses of the magnet, taken from the available extracts out of his works, is worth quoting here :

"There are qualities in a magnet, and one of these qualities is that the magnet also attracts *all martial humours* that are in the human system.

Martial diseases are such as are caused by auras coming and expanding from a centre outwards, and at the same time holding on to their centres; in other words, such as originate from a certain place and extend their influence without leaving the place from which they originate.

In such cases, the magnet should be laid upon the centre, and then it will attract the diseased aura towards the centre, and circumscribe and localise the disease until the latter may be reabsorbed into its centre and, thereby, we may destroy the herd of the virus and cure the patient and we need not wait idly to see what Nature will do.

The magnet, therefore, is very useful in all inflammations, influxes and ulcerations, in diseases of the bowels and uterus, in internal as well as external diseases."

'All martial humours' mean all the liquid or semi-liquid substances of the body which contain iron in any proportion as explained below :

Martial=(L. mars-mart-iron) Pertaining to or containing iron-Syn. Ferruginous.

Humours=(L. fluid) 1. Any fluid or semi-fluid substance in the body.

2. Cardinal humours—Four chief fluids of the body, namely, blood, phlegm, choler (choleratica-bile) and melancholy (black bile).

3. The four juices or fluids recognised in ancient medicine (blood, phlegm, bile and black bile), of which the body was thought to be composed.

Hence the statement of Paracelsus shows that a magnet attracts all the liquid and semi-liquid substances containing even a little quantity of iron and not only blood.

A mixture of the four liquids determines complexions, dispositions, temperaments and physical and mental qualities. The predominance of one of them produces a man who is sanguine, phlegmatic or melancholic and each of them has specific characteristics.

The ancient Unani physicians had formed a theory which explained health and disease on humoral basis. The special features of that theory are also the same for humours, namely blood (*khoon*), phlegm (*balgham*), yellow bile (*safra*) and black bile (*sauda*). This humoralism still holds its position with Unani physicians in India. They believe that when the humours are in proper proportion in respect of their force and quantity, a person enjoys perfect health, but when one or more of them is diminished or increased, the person becomes sick. The characteristics of these four Unani humours are given on following pages.

Humour	Colour and taste	Nature	Type and personality	Functions
Blood (*Khoon*)	Red, sweetish	Hot and wet (*Damwi mizaj*)	Sanguine or plethoric type. Complexion red. Good appetite. Active, tense, obese and robust. Urine reddish.	Provides nutrition to the human body, promotes growth in adolescence, helps in generation of innate heat by supplying fuel to the body.
Phlegm (*Balgham*)	Whitish, can transform into blood	Cold and wet (*Balghami mizaj*)	Phlegmatic type. Drowsy, dull, hair thin, white pasty skin, obese, activities and movements sluggish. Urine colourless ; lack of thirst.	Subserves nutrition to organs like cerebrum, lubricates joints, keeps tissues and organs moist for smooth movement and avoids dryness.
Yellow bile (*Safra*)	Bright red (like, saffron) bitter, light & pungent	Hot and dry (*Safrawi mizaj*)	Choleric or bilious type. Body hairy and lean, complexion sallow. Gets angry quickly, proud and	Enables blood to nourish those organs which need bilious homour (lungs, etc.). Attenuates blood so as to

Humour	Colour and taste	Nature	Type and personality	Functions
			revengeful, energetic; intelligent and shrewd. Sensation of pins and pricks in body. Urine fiery and yellow.	reach the smallest channels of body. Cleanses food residues and phlegmatic humours off the walls of bowels and stimulates intestines. Aids digestion and kills parasites by its bitter taste.
Black bile (*Sauda*)	Dark brown sediment of blood	Cold and dry (*Saudawi mizaj*)	Melancholic type. Dark, thin, with narrow blood vessels, loss of sleep. Urine black or reddish black.	Nourishes some organs (bones) and bestows density and consistency on blood. While travelling to stomach, tickles its mouth and creates a sense of hunger, arousing appetite.

The statement of Paracelsus, therefore, implies that the treatment with magnets has influence on all the humours and on all the persons having any of the above characteristics and thus covers great majority of mankind.

It is a well-known fact that the breath is inhaled cold but exhaled hot, as it passes through hot places. Also, the breath is dry when inhaled and moist when exhaled. If there is loss of heat (hypothermia) or excess of moisture in any person, the constant touch of magnets for some time regulates both as it generates heat in the body.

A pair of magnets has, therefore, multifold benefits. Even if the magnet had only one good quality, it was worth being preserved in every house. But it has so many qualities. In fact, it is a doctor-cum-medicine in itself. It, therefore, becomes imperative that every family must have a pair of magnets and should know how to use it, at least in common ailments of daily occurrence.

India is a poor country and a large number of its people have no money to purchase food or even medicine if they fall sick. Magnetotherapy can very well come to their help in the case of illness at a very little or no cost. Philanthropists can start free 'Magnetotherapy Centres' for free treatment of the poor and needy persons, with a few magnets only, without incurring any high recurring expenditure on medicines or doctors.   ★

13

Magnet as a Preventive Device

Good Health is the Noblest Gift of God

The charter of the World Health Organisation, which works through various Governments, has defined health as : "A state of complete physical, mental and social being, and not merely the absence of disease or infirmities".

Good health is the choicest blessing of life and the noblest gift of God. A man cannot fully enjoy happiness if his health is shaken and life becomes a burden in that case. It is, therefore, the natural and sacred duty of every one to make all possible efforts to preserve good health and to prevent health hazards in future life. Mr. Harvey W. Wiley has so very truly remarked : "We are carefully to preserve that life, which the Author of nature has given us, for it was no idle gift".

The medical science can give us absence of sickness but it cannot give us good health. Others can provide a house for us but they cannot make it a home. Good health, therefore, depends not on services but on self. The self can be protected from so many ills by means of precautions and preventions.

Prevention is Better than Cure

Prevention of disease is definitely better and cheaper than cure, but positive health is better than either. If with healthy housing, sound nutrition, fresh air, and some kind of natural exercise, we can avoid from the very start the conditions which promote many of the modern diseases, we shall not have to face costly treatment for relief, cure and eradication of diseases.

A first class physician is one who could not only cure diseases but could also prevent them. It will not be a good policy

145

to wait till a person becomes ill. To administer medicines for diseases which have already developed and to suppress revolts which have already sprung up, is comparable to the behaviour of those who begin to dig a well after they have become thirsty. It is for this reason that Governments arrange preventive measures against smallpox, etc.

Very often, people are not actually ill, but they feel a little below that they think should be ideal health. This is the pre-clinical stage of disease and due care should be taken at this time to prevent possible disease. If a person is correctly treated at this stage, not only are the unwell feeling and fatigue, etc., cured but he is spared the consequences of developing any serious disease.

Parents who are healthy beget healthy children. The children who are born, healthy, have less diseases in their later lives and enjoy a healthier mental outlook. If adults who were robust as children, become ill, they are easy to cure, but the diseases of the person who were born weakling or who remained ill during the first few years of their lives, are comparatively difficult to cure.

Modern man drinks wine like water, leads an irregular and unnatural life, indulges in sexual excesses and thereby exhausts his vital force. He is wasting his energy excessively and is seeking only physical pleasures. All these actions are against the rules of nature. Hence, people reach only half the age of hundred years stipulated in ancient religious books and begin to degenerate. Keeping one's habits regular and taking some natural exercise is necessary for one to live in health for a long time.

Descartes (1596—1650), a great Astronomer and Philosopher said : "If there is any possible means of increasing the common wisdom and ability of mankind it must be sought in medicine". Indeed so, as medicine is the "Science of Humanity and Life". Here we are reminded of the views of Dr. F.V. Broussais of France, who said : "If magnetism is true, medicine would be an absurdity". And it has been proved, beyond doubt, by a large number of scientists, through so many experiments all over the world, that magnetism is a true science. According to these great personalities, therefore, all benefits in the matter of health and wisdom should be derived from the use of magnetism.

Use of Magnet as a Preventive Device

Let us now discuss the use of magnet as a preventive device. It is seen that when some danger to existence is impending, man, by instinct, either runs away from it or raises barriers to bar its approach. But man cannot run away from a disease creeping in his own physical self. He can only create internal and external safeguards against the impending illness. Safeguards of both types aim at increasing resistance in the body. The resistance can be created through two means :

(a) By cleansing the body of any undesirable accumulations, removing obstacles and regularising the working of the human machinery; and

(b) By providing new vigour and stimulation to the energies in the body.

Magnet is capable of doing the wonderful job of accomplishing both the above objectives. Thus magnet proves a strong safeguard against illness and serves as a highly beneficial preventive device.

In homoeopathic system of treatment, curative remedies are given for preventive purposes also. Similarly, the use of magnet is equally rewarding in both the ways. This is so because magnetotherapy works on the principle of accelerating the innate (not the superficial) resistance and dynamism in the body.

Magnetotherapy rejects the practice of injecting foreign agents or elements into the body to do fighting with the disease. Hence preventive or precautionary application of magnet is essentially beneficial and devoid of any harmful effects.

It can be safely said regular application of magnets of advised power is capable of substituting the morning and evening excrcises in at least the physical domain. Psychological and natural benefits accruing from exercises cannot and should not, of course, be ignored, especially by the youth, but the use of magnet could be an additional aid to the healthy and the most valuable assistance for persons of advancing and advanced age. Hence healthy persons are advised regular or frequent use of magnets for preserving and improving upon their existing state of health—especially those who cannot spare time for any other exercise or walking.

We have seen, in Chapter 8, how magnets work on the human body. The magnet works in various ways but the main action is through the blood circulatory system. If our blood is kept clean from deposits and impurities, we shall be saved from a large number of ailments which may otherwise afflict us. And this object can be achieved by the use of magnets. Their use proves curative in the case of sick persons, restorative in the case of convalescents and preventive in the case of healthy persons.

The magnetism of the human body need to be regularly strengthened by external feeding if proper health is to be maintained. All the constituents and internal systems of our body naturally respond to the magnetic emanations and invariably show positive results. Magnetic flux invigorates and accelerates the self-curative and self-healing agents in the body. Through its action on blood, nerves, cells and hormones, it dynamically adds to the physical, mental and consequently psychological energies of man, fights out exhaustion and sickness and prolongs life. Therefore, application of magnet is bound to contribute towards preservation of health and activity and prevention of impending diseases.

Application of Magnet—Curative as well as Preventive

The application of magnet has its penetrating effect on all the systems working in the human body. Hence it is beneficial for all the ailments and functional defects appearing in the body. And for whatever ailments it can prove useful as curative, it can also prove advantageous as preventive.

In view of the manifold beneficial effects of the magnetic treatment, curative as well as preventive, let us act according to the advice of Dr. R.S. Thacker, a great magnetotherapist of Delhi, in the following verse :

Take two magnets, different pole,
Touch them daily, make a goal.

In short, the matter given so far in all the previous pages has amply shown that the regular user of a pair of magnets stays younger and lives longer. Thus he gets maximum results with minimum efforts, expense and time.

Part VI

14

Experiences of Indian Magnetotherapists

Cases treated by the Author and Others

Magnetotherapy is considered to be a new system of treatment although it is not so as we have seen in Chapter 2. The oldest Magnetotherapist in India in the present times, as far as the Author knows, is Dr. R.S. Thacker of Delhi, He is a businessman but has been giving quite free magnetic treatment for three hours in the morning everyday for the last 20 years. He has cured many thousands of patients of different diseases— acute as well as chronic—hundreds of whom are considered hopeless and were given up as lost by doctors and hospitals. It is not possible to give a long list of these cases treated successfully in this book. However, some 25 cases taken at random are given below for the information of the readers.

Some Cases treated by Dr. R.S. Thacker, Kashi Ram Building, Kashi Ram Lane, Dareeba Kalan, Delhi-110006.

1. *Eczema*—Shri K.C. Gupta (about 52), a high official of the Government of India, New Delhi, was once looking after some flower plants in his bungalow. He got a prick of a thorn on the back of his palm. A few days later, a pimple arose at the point of the prick and took a turn into weeping eczema. The eczema spread to the whole of his body and discharge began to ooze out of every limb. The doctors of the Government dispensaries, including Skin specialists, tried to cure his eczema but nobody could even relieve him. The disease made his life miserable and no system of treatment seemed to help him. He was then advised to try Magnetotherapy. He approached Dr. Thacker and started taking his treatment. He was treated by

153

methods I and V alternately with strong magnets for 10 minutes once daily in the morning. His wounds began to dry up in 3-4 days and he was cured of his horrible, eczematic disease in about three weeks, without any medicine.

It was this surprising cure that created a desire in the author to learn this wonderful system of treatment, for the benefit of the public in general.

2. *Accident*—Shri Avinash Kumar Shukla, Delhi had met with an accident when the former's motor cycle collided against a car. He suffered from acute intolerable pain but after magnetic treatment given to him, he got complete relief. He could sleep comfortably because his pain had gone and he could recover at a very swift rate. The very next day he went to his shop and worked there, although stitches were there. He could walk straight and felt as if he was not at all injured.

3. *Accident*—Rajeev Jain, a student of Delhi, met with an accident while playing cricket and got his lower lip injured about 6 milli-metres inside his mouth. He was cured completely and made perfectly alright with magnetic treatment within a period of 3 days of the accident. He wrote afterwards that magnetic treatment was really a magic treatment that he had so far seen.

4. *Arthritis of Knees*—The wife of Shri L.D. Gupta, M.A., Shahdara, was a patient of arthritis of knees for some time. Her disease rendered the movement of her legs very painful and she felt great difficulty in getting up and walking about. Long Allopathic and the Unani treatment were of hardly any benefit to her. She started undergoing magnetic treatment and responded to it very well. The short course given to her brought her considerable relief from pain and numbness of limbs.

5. *Burns*—Dr. Thacker's sister-in-law, wife of a Sessions Judge at Simla, got very severe burns on the right side of her breast. She had suppurated wounds and could not sleep on account of pain in the wounds. The best Allopathic treatment available at Simla could not cure her. Dr. Thacker went to

Simla, with some strong magnets, and treated her there. He applied two magnets to her hands for two sittings of 15 minutes each. She felt the action of the magnets on her body but there was no relief to her wounds. Dr. Thacker then hanged a magnet from the roof of her room, made her sit on a wooden chair and asked her to hold the magnet in close contact with the wounds, twice daily, for 15 minutes each time. After a few days' treatment, the wounds dried up and she was relieved of her serious painful trouble. The magnet was hanged from the roof so that the patient might not feel the weight of the magnet on the wounds.

6. *Chorea (Parkinsonism)*—Shri Brindaban Sharma (about 60) had chorea in his hands. His hands used to suffer from involuntary motions for 8-10 years. He was given treatment under method I, once daily in morning. He was cured of his chronic disease in about a month's time.

7. *Diabetes*—(*i*) Shri Sharma (about 45) was suffering from diabetes. He approached Dr. Thacker for Magnetotherapy and was treated by method No. I. During the course of the treatment, he had to go to Kashmir. He took two magnets from Dr. Thacker and used them there. When he came back after about 2 months, he said that his diabetes had been cured and he returned the magnets.

(*ii*) Shri Sharma's father (70-75 years old) was also suffering from diabetes. He also took magnetic treatment, by method No. I, and got well in about two months.

8. *Fits after Injury*—A girl of 20-21 years was getting fits and sometimes became unconscious, since the age of 5-6 years, when she had a fall from the roof of a house. She was given magnetic treatment by method I. In two months' period her fits became very few, say once a week instead of once every day and in another two-three months she was quite free from her fits and occasional unconsciousness.

9. *Hernia*—A lady (about 40) was suffering from umbilical hernia. Allopathic doctors advised operation but she was afraid

of it and wanted to avoid it. She, therefore, took magnetic treatment. Four powerful magnets were applied simultaneously. Two were applied to her feet under method No. V, a third magnet (North pole) to her abdomen over the navel and the fourth magnet (South pole) to her back. She was cured of her disease in about three months' period without any medicine or operation.

10. *Hiccup (Hi cough)*—An elderly lady brought her newly married daughter-in-law to Dr. Thacker for treatment. The girl was suffering from occasional hiccough for many years. The elderly lady said that if she knew about the girl's disease, she would not have married her son with her. Dr. Thacker assured both of them that the girl would be cured of her disease. He applied North pole of a strong magnet to the upper part of her navel and South pole of another magnet, just opposite to it, on the back, once daily in the morning. The girl was cured of her disease in about a week's time.

11. *A Hopeless Case*—Mistri Zia-uddin used to work in Dr. Thacker's workshop of silverware. Zia-uddin's mother was seriously ill ; all hopes of her survival had been given up and relatives gathered to witness her end and to do the needful thereafter. Zia-uddin told everything to Dr. Thacker and took him to his house. Two magnets were applied to her by method II. She passed a large stool with very bad intolerable, stinking smell and she felt better immediately thereafter. After some time, she went to her native place at Moradabad instead of going to graveyard in Delhi.

12. *Injury in Legs*—Shri C.R. (55), met with an accident in front of his shop and got injured. He was given indigenous medicines and was later placed under Allopathic treatment but was not cured thereby. He had pain in his legs all the time. He came limping to Dr. Thacker's clinic. He was treated with magnets (method V.). He started feeling the effect of the magnets after about 30 minutes and continued the treatment upto 90 minutes. He felt so much relief by this treatment that he went back walking almost like a normal man. He, however, continued the treatment for some time more.

13. *Another Injury*—Dr. Thacker's younger brother (about 40) once fell down from the front seat of a tonga and got hurt in his right leg badly. There was no fracture but it became very difficult for him to walk about. He, however, managed to reach his brother's clinic somehow. Dr. Thacker first applied a pair of magnets of medium strength to his feet for 45 minutes. After 15 minutes, he applied two strong magnets, which could lift more than 20 kg. of iron-weight, on the spots of injury, for about one hour. The pain and swelling subsided very soon and no medicine was required to be given to him.

14. *Menses Absent*—A girl of 21 years had no menses at all. She was treated by Dr. Thacker by placing two strong round encased magnets, *both having South Pole*, in her hands. The treatment continued for 20-25 days. The girl had her first menses and her menses were quite regular thereafter. He advises that in such cases both magnets should have the same pole in the centre, preferably South Pole.

15. *Mental Retardation*—A child (12 years) of New Delhi, was mentally retarded. A medium power magnet was applied to his forehead for 5 minutes daily and magnetised water was given for drinking. The treatment continued for 3 months and the boy became quite normal in this period.

16. *Mental Sickness*—Sardar B.S. (27 years) could not do any mental work. He preferred to remain silent, talked rarely and became unconscious sometimes. He took magnetic treatment for about 6 months and drank magnetised water during the whole treatment. He became not only normal but over-active and is now running his business successfully.

17. *Obesity*—(i) The betrothal of a young girl was delayed on account of her obesity. She took magnetic treatment. She lost her weight by about 4 kgs. in about 2 months and her marriage was settled.

(ii) A milk-vendor of Delhi (about 55 years) had almost double the weight of a normal male of his age. He felt difficulty in doing his work and in walking. He took magnetic treatment. Two strong magnets were applied to his hands, other two to his soles and a fifth one on the lowest part of his spine—all five simultaneously. Treatment was started from 10 minutes and the time was increased by 5 minutes every day up to 45 minutes per sitting. He lost much weight and became active in one month. He purchased two strong magnets and applied them at home for about 4 months. In this period, he shed off so much of his excess flesh and weight that some people could not recognise him sometimes.

18. *Pain in Arm*—Dr. Thacker once got severe pain in the upper part of his right arm. He applied South pole of a strong magnet on the place of pain. The pain drifted to a lower point near the elbow He applied the magnet on the paining portion near the elbow. The pain drifted further lower to his wrist. He moved the magnet to his wrist. The pain went up to the upper arm again. He followed the pain with the magnet there also. Then the pain left him completely. All this happened in one day only and the pain did not recur thereafter.

19. *Pain in Back*—A boy (about 10) was suffering from severe pain in his spine below the neck for about two weeks and was crying almost all the time. The boy was brought to Dr. Thacker for treatment. The South pole of a magnet was applied to the paining spot for 15 minutes. The pain moved to another place. The magnet was also shifted to the new pain spot. In about half an hour, the pain vanished and the boy began to smile. The child went back from the clinic talking and smiling while he was brought in his father's lap in crying mood.

20. *Paralysis*—A girl of about 4 years, was suffering from paralysis. She was brought in lap by his father. Treatment was given to her by methods I and V, 10 minutes daily, along with magnetic water. The disease had afflicted her for about 8-10 days only. She recovered fully from her disease in about a month's time.

21. *Polio* (*i*)—A girl aged over one year got an attack of Polio. She got treated in Kalawati Saran Hospital and at other places but to no avail. In the end, he got her treated

by Dr R.S. Thacker with the magnets and she became alright, he could go to school herself. The treatment worked as a wonder in her case.

(*ii*)—Miss Barkha, Delhi, had an attack of Polio. She was treated by many doctors but to no progress. Then she was kept under the treatment of Dr R.S. Thacker which made her hale and hearty.

22. *Pulmonary Tuberculosis*—Smt. D.S. (40), Delhi, was suffering from tuberculosis of lungs. She was so weak that she could not sit on a bench without support. The usual symptoms of cough, fever, phlegm, etc., were there. Doctors had declared her a hopeless case. She was given treatment by method No.I for 10 minutes, along with magnetised water three to four times a day. As she could not attend Dr. Thacker's Clinic every day her son used to take magnets home and apply them there. In about two months, she become alright and appetite increased. She later got checked up by the T.B. Clinic and they declared that no trace of T.B. was left in her body.

23. *Unable to Move*—Smt. S. D. (70) attended a Devi Jagran, throughout one night, at the second storey of a house. At the time of Arti in early morning, her feet became benumbed and she could neither walk nor stand. Her sons brought her down as she could not stand on her legs. She was brought to Dr. Thacker. He applied strong magnets to her feet (method V). After the application of the magnets for about 90 minutes, she was able not only to stand on her legs but also to walk without any support. She did not get any trouble later and no further treatment was required.

24. *Skin Disease*—Shri R. Aggarwal, Delhi, had been suffering from some skin disease for the last 7-8 years which remained uncured inspite of his having consulted the best skin specialist. He then took magnetic treatment from Dr. R.S. Thacker. He was amazed to see the convincing result within 10 days only in which he felt great relief and was quite free from the trouble within that short period.

25. *Throat Trouble*—Shri V.K. Nayyar, wrote in his letter to Dr. Thacker that his mother Smt. Rajinder Pal Nayyar had got some trouble with her throat and she almost stopped speaking. She had been given every kind of treatment namely; Allopathic, Homoeopathic and Ayurvedic but all in vain. So he approached Dr. Thacker for some treatment to be given to his mother and Dr. Thacker arranged for some magnetic treatment for her. He had added that after few days' treatment she was alright and was speaking perfectly normal.

Dr. Thacker has increased the height of many girls and boys of young age by 2 to 3 cms. with application of magnets and giving magnetised water to drink. He has also done it in the case of some girls of marriageable age and some young males.

Dr. R.S. Thacker also rendered free humanitarian service towards treatment of the jawans hospitalised in the Military Hospital, Delhi Cantt., through Magnetotherapy, for a period of 6 months during 1971-72, just after the last war with Pakistan. He effected very appreeiable cures in the hospital and became popular among the inmates there.

SOME OF THE CASES TREATED BY THE AUTHOR

I have got the best success with application of magnets in Cervical Spondylitis—(Inflammation and pain of any of the cervical vertebrae of the spinal cord). It becomes difficult to move the neck sideways or up and down and all movements are painful. There is no good or permanent treatment in Allopathic system of treatment or in other systems for this disease. The hospitals give diathermy, traction, wax bath, physiotherapy and sometimes ultra-sonic rays and suggest neck collars. But all of these treatments give the patients only temporary relief for a few hours or for a few days and the trouble returns thereafter. Patients continue taking these treatments in hospitals for years together but seldom get permanent cure.

The disease generally occurs as a result of wrong posture of sitting and doing table work for long hours with bent neck and upper part of the back on any one side. The pain extends to right shoulder and right arm sometimes and to left shoulder and left arm in some other cases. In some cases, it goes even to lumbar region (tail end of the spine cord). It seldom troubles the labour class people or the persons who do a lot of physical exercise of the whole body. It is, therefore, said to be a disease of well-to-do people but it is very troublesome and inconvenient for those who unfortunately get it.

As I have got more than 95% success in this disease, I would start stating my cases with this disease only.

Some Cases of Cervical Spondylitis

Technique of Treatment

My procedure has been that I get the cervical region of the patient X-rayed with a view to ascertain as to which particular vertebrae are affected in that case. Generally, any consequtive two or three vertebrae are affected but in some cases more vertebrae up to five may be affected.

I apply the North pole of the High Power Magnet on the affected vertebrae and South pole to the place up to which the pain extends—irrespective of whether it goes to right side or left side or even to the lumbar region. Both the magnets are applied simultaneously for about 10-12 minutes. In chronic cases, the time may be gradually increased by one minute every day up to 20 minutes. The same treatment can be given in the evening also if required.

The intake of cold drinks and eatables which produce cold effect and gas in the body should be avoided.

1. Shri S.K.B. (45 years), a Govt. official, had been suffering from this disease for two years. He had pain in the left side of the cervical region of his spine, in the left shoulder and in the left arm. He could not lift or move his left arm freely. He had taken the best available Allopathic treatment. physiotherapy and

traction treatment, without permanent relief. He took magnetic treatment for about a month and got rid of his ailment. He is perfectly alright now.

2.   Mrs. P.G. Gokhale, New Delhi, was suffering from Spondylitis for about two years. She did not get sleep due to pain and there was no free movement of hands particularly her left arm. She underwent magnet-treatment for about 35 days in February—March 1976. Her husband was glad to certify that the aforesaid treatment gave her complete relief.

3.   Shri B.D. Nagpal, New Delhi, a youngman of 40 years was suffering from pain in neck, left shoulder and back since 1972. He was admitted to A.I.I.M.S. Hospital for about three weeks and was under their treatment for about $1\frac{1}{2}$ years. But no relief. He then contacted this Centre and took magnet-treatment and felt almost completely cured.

4.   Shri K.P. Agarwal, New Delhi, Representative and Liaison Officer of a large number of big companies of Bombay got pain in his left shoulder extending to left arm and causing much inconvenience all time especially in lifting his arm or taking bath. He consulted the heart specialist and the Hony. Physician to the President of India who diagnosed the disease to be cervical spondylitis. Mr. Agarwal had heard that there was no good treatment under modern medicine for this disease and that magnets have cured many patients of this disease. He, therefore, took magnet-treatment for about two weeks and this treatment cured him of his painful condition completely without any side effect.

5.   Dr. Gulsan R. Virmani, M.B.B.S., F.R.C.S., D.C.G. (England) New Delhi, was suffering from Prolapse Intervertebral Disc for about one year. The pain used to be very severe. The conservative modern treatment given for this condition did not help him at all. Eventually, he discussed this case with me. I advised him

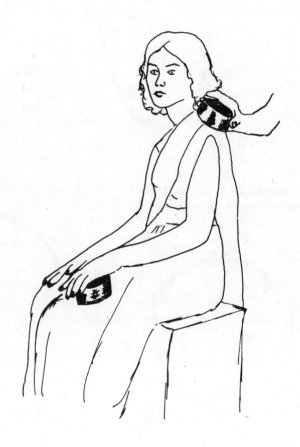

Treatment for CERVICAL SPONDYLITIS:
North Pole of High Power Magnets on affected Cervical Vertebrae and
South Pole on the spot upto which the pain extends.

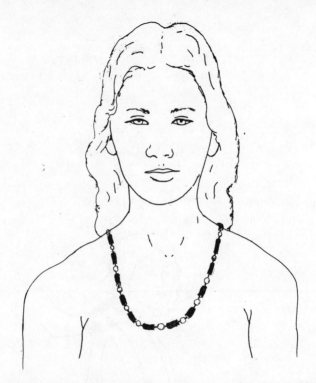

Magnetic Necklace: For ailment of neck and chest. Wearing the Necklace with Magnets touching the affected part.

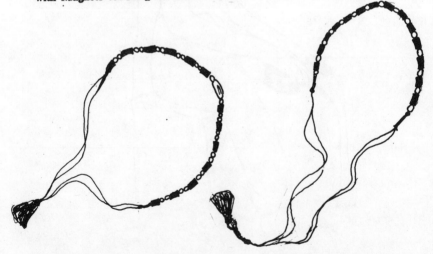

MAGNETIC NECKLACES: Made with small Ceramic Magnets and silver chain or Nylon thread, used for Asthma, Bronchitis, Chest ailments etc...

Silver Necklace: Contains 20 small magnets in silver chain, like a beautiful

to try magnetotherapy for a few days. This, of course, he did for about a fortnight. He was more than glad to say after that period that he was quite pain-free then.

6. Maj. D.S. Cheema—Delhi Cantt—aged 45 years was suffering from cervical spondylitis for the last 4 years. He applied magnets for two months. He started feeling improvement after three weeks and got 90% cured in two months. There remained no pain or stiffness in his neck region.

There are several other cases of cervical spondylitis who have come to this Centre and have been completely cured within a month or two. Some of them took Homoeopathic medicine also along with the magnet-treatment while others did not. The success mentioned above is doubly appreciable as the method of modern medicine has no effective cure for this disease. I would like to content myself with giving only a few cases of this disease as well as of some other diseases in these pages so that the readers of the book can be convinced that Magnetotherapy can do great service in many kinds of functional disorders and diseases.

There is another kind of spondylitis called 'Ankylosing Spondylitis'. This is quite different from Cervical Spondylitis and is not amenable to any treatment easily. Magnetotherapy can help persons suffering from this disease also to some extent, as far as the pains, swellings and stiffness of their parts is concerned but it is difficult for any system to cure them completely without divine help.

Appendicitis

7. Kumari U.M. (40 years) had pain in the region of her appendix. The South pole of a strong encased magnet was applied to the painful part for 10-15 minutes daily for a few days and the pain subsided gradually. It was completely removed in about 4-5 days.

Asthma

8. Mr. Pramod Prakash Tyagi, New Delhi—writes that he has been suffering from Asthma for the last 15 years. He began to feel the effect of Asthma right from the beginning of October-November each year and he had to remain engulfed in this disease throughout the winter season. In the year 1977, he started using magnets for some benefit in this disease with my advice and continued the treatment regularly with the result that he had no attack of Asthma throughout the winter. He says that he has felt a peculiar feeling in his body, as a result of magnet-treatment, that there was a special kind of activity in his body throughout the season, He was astonished to see this effect of magnet-treatment in his body.

9. Smt. Ganga Devi, aged about 56 years, had been suffering from Asthma for the last 25 years, from serious headache for six years and from severe pain in her knees for the last 2-3 years. She used the magnets for three months. All her troubles almost vanished. She arranged to obtain a pair of magnets and used them as a precautionery measure every now and then so that she may not get any of these or any other ailment in her old age.

10. A youngman of 27 years R.R. Bahl used to get Asthmatic attacks in the beginning of every summer with the result that he had to take leave from his office in April and May every year. He started taking magnet-treatment in March, 1978 and continued it for a few months. The treatment had such a good effect on him that he did not get even a single attack throughout the summer in 1978 and he did not take even a single day's leave from office. He used to touch the high-powered magnets with his palms for 10 minutes once in 24 hours.

Boils

11. Shri R., a teacher (45 years), got recurring boils in his buttocks for six months. He got them operated twice but in vain. Even after the operations, more boils cropped up, causing pain and obstructions in his sitting in a chair or riding a bicycle. He was given magnetic treatment in his soles. Some boils burst while some others subsided and he was completely cured of his extremely painful disease in 3 months.

12. Shri P.D. Srivastava, M.Sc., D. Phil, Entomologist, New Delhi, had come to know about Magnetotherapy through MORNING ECHO, Hindustan Times publication, and tried this therapy on several members of his family as follows :

    (a) First of all his wife used magnets for her Sciatica pain from which she had been suffering for the last 4 years. She used the magnets for 4 months and was fully cured.

    (b) His daughter aged 24 years had been using spectacles for the last 4 years. She used the magnets for 6 months, after that she left using spectacles.

    (c) His second daughter aged 14 years was suffering from Rheumatic pain in her right hip joints for the last 2 years. She started magnet-treatment towards the end of May 1977. When she found that magnet-treatment is useful, she obtained a pair of magnets. She could use the magnets later on also. Now she is not having any rheumatic pain.

    A few months back she had leucodermic patches in her right hand she found distinct improvement in the patches also, by the use of the magnets.

    (d) His eldesh son used the magnets whenever he got headache and he got relief within a few minutes.

Eczema

13. Shri P.S.K., a Supreme Court Advocate (48 years), had

eczema on his feet for the past 35-36 years. Originally his eczema was weeping but it became dry for some years. There was itching, burning, unevenness and blackishness of skin when he started magnetic treatment. He was given this treatment in his soles for 10 minutes each day for about $1\frac{1}{2}$ months. Itching and burning completely subsided from all the diseased parts and the skin of his feet became smooth and less blackish. His progress was extremely satisfactory in this short time.

14. Late Shri Suraj Narain, New Delhi, was suffering from eczema in his feet for more than 2 years. He was under the treatment of skin specialist. A senior doctor told him that there was no cure for eczema in Allopathy. He was advised to try magnetotherapy and he contacted this Centre. He was completely cured of the eczema except that the skin on the feet remained a bit rough.

15. Shri N. Krishnamurthy, New Delhi-21, brought his wife who had been suffering from eczema in her right palm for 3 years. She took all modern treatments but in vain. He read about magnet-treatment in the Times of India. He approached this Centre, with the zero hope. She was however advised to try magnet-treatment for a fortnight. She actually began to feel better in about two weeks. She took the treatment regularly for two months and was completely cured. Later on he sent several patients to this Centre for treatment with magnets.

16. Shri S.S. Madan, New Delhi, was suffering from very bad type of eczema in an area of 16 sq. inches in his left foot & leg since 1958. Pus used to ooze out of the wounds and there was intense itching all the time which resulted in bleeding sometimes. His life had become miserable and he thought that his disease was incurable. He tried all known systems of treatment but to

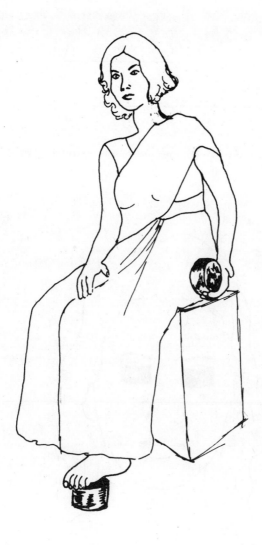

Left-sided Sciatica: North Pole on the left hip and South Pole under left sole. Similar application may be made on the right side for Right sided Sciatica.

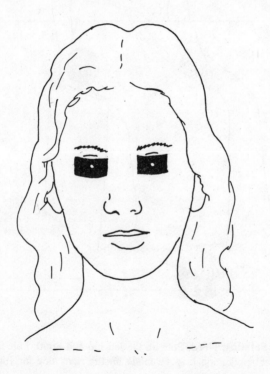

Ceramic Magnets on the Eyes: For eye ailments such as pain, redness, watering, swelling, initial stages of Cataract and for improving vision.

no use. He started magnetic treatment in May 1977. This treatment had a miraculous effect on his eczema and all his wounds were dried up. During magnetic treatment, he did not use any medicine internally or externally. Hence he could definitely say that the recovery was due only to the magnetic treatment. He calls magnetic treatment a boon for disappointed patients suffering from chronic diseases.

Eye Trouble

17. Shri Suresh Prakash, Delhi-110007, writes that his wife, Smt. Kiran Kumari, aged 37, had been suffering from different sorts of eye troubles for about 2 years and she felt weakness in her eyes. Doctor advised her to wear glasses of a very high number. The glasses were got made and she began to use them. Meanwhile, he contacted this Centre. She was given a pair of Ceramic Magnets to apply on her both eyes. To the surprise of the family, she felt tremendous relief within a week and left using glasses. All sorts of eye troubles were gone. Now she could read newspapers at night even, which was previously difficult for her to do.

Goitre

18. A young girl, Km. B.B. (20 years), had goitre for about one year. She took magnetic treatment for about 4 months regularly. Two strong magnets were applied to her hands and two other crescent type ceramic magnets were applied to the swollen thyroid gland, each pair for about 10 minutes daily. The hardness of the swelling was removed and the size of the goitre was considerably reduced. She had to discontinue the treatment on account of her marriage.

Headache

19. Shri Radhey Shyam, Delhi-110051, was suffering from headache on the right side for the last 5 years. His agony, pain, anxiety and suffering can beter be

understood than described because no treatment was benefitting him. He was also feeling kidney weakness due to prolonged suffering. He, therefore, took magnet-treatment by applying small magnets on the head and high powered magnets under the feet. He found much improvement in his health and his ailments almost disappeared.

Hernia

20.   A male child of about 10 months was suffering from hernia of left side. Sometimes the intestine used to protrude out of the level of abdomen when the child felt some inconvenience and at some other times it went back to its normal position. The South pole of the crescent type ceramic magnet was applied locally on the place of hernia for 5 to 10 minutes in the morning. After about one month, there was no protrusion and, therefore, no inconvenience to the child.

Injury

21.   Dr. M.T.S. (35 years) met with an accident while boarding a bus and severely sprained his left foot. He was unable to walk due to unbearable pain and swelling. The South pole of a strong encased magnet was applied for about 20 minutes. After two such applications he was greatly relieved of his pain and swelling and was able to move about almost normally.

Insomnia (Due to Injury)

22.   Shri P.D. (60 years) met with a serious accident and the whole of his right leg was plastered in a Hospital. He had much pain and could not sleep at night. A magnet was applied to his forehead at about 10 P.M. for about 20 minutes daily for some days. He started getting sleep and could sleep well after a few days.

Lachrymation from One Eye

23.   Smt. P.D. (40 years) had lachrymation from her right eye only, for two years, without any apparent cause.

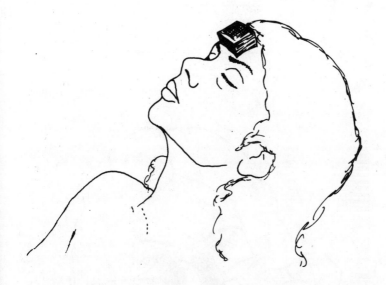

South Pole of Ceramic Magnets on the Forehead: Used for inducing sleep, half an hour before going to bed.

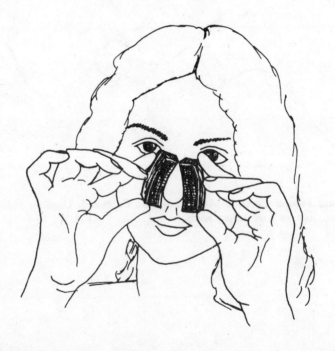

For Diseases of Nose: Namely constant cold, sneezing, watering, polypus, blockage, sinusitis, etc. Apply Ceramic Magnets on both Nostrils. North Pole on the right Nostril and South Pole on the left Nostril for 10 minutes twice daily.

A strong encased magnet was applied to her right palm and a small round magnet was applied to her watering eye. She continued this treatment for about $1\frac{1}{2}$ months and the watering of her eye stopped completely.

Menses Improved

24. Smt. J.K. (40 years) used to come for treatment of her backache, which was troubling her for years. She was given treatment with 2 strong encased magnets in her soles every evening. After about 15 days she reported that she not only felt better in respect of her backache but also got better and satisfactory menses after the magnet-treatment.

Nasal Polypus

25. Mrs. Gauri Shankar Lakhotia, Delhi, had nasal polypus and enlargement of bone in both of her nostrils with the result that she found difficulty in breathing. She used to get up and sit up at night and begin to sneeze which resulted in the flow of much water and great inconvenience at night. Allopathic and Ayurvedic treatment was given to her but they did not cure her. Lastly, doctors advised operation which she did not agree to. She started magnet-treatment at this Centre. Gradually the fleshy growth and enlargement of bone in her nose began to shrink. On the opening of the nostrils the difficulty in breathing was gradually removed and she became completely free from the trouble.

Obesity

26. Mrs. Joginder Kaur, New Delhi. Her height was 157 cms, weight 66 kgs. She started taking magnetic treatment in this Centre for reducing her weight from 3rd June 1977 and continued it till 2nd July, 1977 regularly. Her weight was reduced to 62 kgs. and she did not feel any weakness or tiredness, rather she felt more activeness and freshness. If she felt tired on account of working during the day, the tiredness

was also removed on her using the magnets in the evening. She used to apply the magnets only once in 24 hours for 10 minutes in the evening—5 minutes under the palms and 5 minutes under the soles. She felt that the effect of magnetic treatment remained in the body even after leaving the treatment.

(This was a case of unusual reduction of weight in a month's time. Everyone does not lose weight at this rate. But every-body who takes this treatment loses 1 to 2 pounds every month for a few months).

27.   Km. S.M. 20 years—Height 1.5 m., weight 65 kg.—took magnetic treatment for 20 days and lost her weight by ½ kg. She could not continue the treatment as she had to go out of station.

28.   Km. A.S., 16 years—Height 1.65 m., weight 70 kg.—took magnetic treatment for one month and lost weight by 1/2 kg. She also could not continue the treatment on account of unavoidable circumstances.

In both these cases treatment was given by applying one set of strong magnets to hands and another set of magnets to feet simultaneously. The magnets reduce the excess flesh and therefore the excess weight of the body without reducing activity, alertness and strength. No dieting is necessary with this system of treatment.

Orchitis

29.   A boy of 6 years was suffering from inflammation of right testis with scrotal enlargement for a few years. The scrotum had unusual shine and abnormal crimson colour and was hanging down about 2.5 cm longer than the left one. Doctors had advised operation but his parents wanted to avoid it. The South pole of a crescent type magnet was applied to the enlarged scrotum daily for 15 minutes for about 6 months. The size of the scrotum was reduced by about three-fourths and normal skin colour was restored.

Pain in Arm

30. A girl of about 10 years was brought by her mother
for treatment of severe intolerable pain in her left arm.
The South pole of a strong encased magnet was applied
to the paining part and the pain was completely relieved
by this local treatment in about 15 minutes.

Pain in Finger

31. Late Dr. T.N.G., Homoeopath (65 years) had pain in
the first finger of his right hand, without any apparent
cause. The South pole of a bar magnet was applied to
his finger 3-4 times daily for 10 minutes each time,
The pain vanished in 2-3 days.

Pain in Hand

32. A young lady of 24-25 years suddenly got unbearable
pain between her right thumb and first finger. She held
her right hand in her left hand when she came and
could not hang it down. Her face showed much agony
and she was in tears. The afflicted portion was kept
in between two magnets—North and South poles. She
was completely cured of the intolerable pain in 15
minutes and went back smiling.

Pain in Jaw

33. Smt. T. (55 years) had severe pain and stiffness around
her right jaw-bone for several years. The pain extended to her right ear and up to head. She was unable
to open her mouth properly and felt great difficulty
in eating. The condition had come about after extraction of three teeth and she was treated by many eminent doctors without beneficial results. The South pole
of a bar magnet was applied at the site of the pain for 15
minutes daily and a strong encased magnet was applied
once a week. After about 1½ months of this treatment,
she was completely relieved of all her trouble.

Pain in Knee

34. Pt. S.N. Sharma (78 years) had a fall in a drain and

was suffering from pain in his right knee for three months. The South pole of a small round cylindrical magnet was tied to his knee for half-an-hour daily for 3 days. His pain decreased gradually and vanished completely on the 4th day.

Psoriasis

35. Km. V.K. (24 years) was suffering from Psoriasis for the past 16 years. She got this disease at the age of 8 years after an injection for seasonal boils. She had patches of raw skin of the diameter of about one cm all over her body (except face). Sometimes scales formed and peeled off. All kinds of treatment had been tried but in vain. She took magnetic treatment for about one month. Most of the small patches disappeared and the size of the others greatly shrank, although she was not able to take this treatment regularly.

36. Smt. Subhadra Singhal, New Delhi. She got Psoriasis in her foot which spread to other parts of her body, namely, head, back, hands and feet within two months. She was in great trouble on account of this disease. She was bed-ridden for several months and took several kinds of treatment during this period. She was told that magnetic treatment had good effect on skin diseases and she started using magnets. She began feeling better after some time to the extent that the whole Psoriasis vanished. This effect is a sort of wonder of magnets.

Rheumatism

37. Smt. K.M. (62 years) had rheumatic pain in both her knees and could hardly walk. Two strong magnets were applied to her feet for 15 minutes daily. After a treatment of about 2 months, she was cured of her pain, stiffness and lameness.

38. Mrs. Kamala Ghosh—New Delhi, aged 50 years, was suffering from rheumatic and sciatica pain for about 12 years. She used magnets on her knee, waist and other parts and continued this treatment for three months and all her pains were gone. Even after two years, she did not get the pains again.

Severe Toothache

39. Smt. V. (33 years) had pain in her teeth for 6 years. One evening the pain became unbearable and she decided to get 5-6 teeth extracted next morning. Her husband brought her for some medicine so that she could sleep for some hours during that night Crescent-type ceremic magnets were applied to her jaw from outside. She was advised to continue magnet-treatment and to postpone extraction for 3 days. She agreed and took magnet-treatment for 15 minutes every evening. In 3 days, she got so well that she abandoned the idea of extraction of her teeth. She continued the magnet-treatment for about a month after which there was no pain in her teeth at all.

Stiffness of Neck

40. Km. P.A. (15 years) felt pain and stiffness in her neck one morning. She went to school as usual. When she returned, the pain was severe and was gradually increasing. It became unbearable in the evening and she could not move her neck. She was in tears when she came for treatment. The South pole of a magnet was applied to her neck for half an hour. The pain and stiffness were relieved to a great extent. She was completely cured of her pain and stiffness in the second sitting next morning.

Stomach Acidity and Gas Formation

41. Cap. Ragbhir Singh, New Delhi, was suffering from stomach acidity and gas formation for 7 years. He tried Allopathic enzymes, Homoeopathic remedies and

Ayurvedic medicines but to no effect. He started
magnetic treatment in this Centre. In about a month's
treatment, 75% trouble   vanished. In addition to
magnetic touch, he was given magnetised water to
drink which further improved his condition. He felt
the magnetic treatment to be some sort of *Jadu* Treatment.

Swelling in Knee

42.   Shri T.C.J. (56 years) had swelling and pain in his
knees for 3-4 months. A round cylindrical magnet was
tried to his knee at night and it remained on his knee
throughout the night. The swelling and pain both left
his knee after about a fortnight.

Tiredness and General Weakness

43.   Mr. Balkrishan Agarwal, Lucknow, had come to Delhi
for business and stayed with me. In the evening he
felt extremely tired on account of heavy working
during the day. He felt as if the whole room was
rotating. I gave him two magnets to keep under his
feet. After 15 minutes, his whole tiredness was gone
and he felt quite fresh. The next day also he felt very
tired on account of heavy work and got tired. He was
again given two magnets next day also and he had the
same effect that day as well.

Tonsils

44.   The crescent-type ceramic magnets are beneficial for
removing irritation, pain and swelling of tonsils and
mumps. They are also useful in cough arising from
throat as well as in reducing the swellings of glands
around neck. A number of cases of tonsillitis have
been cured by this treatment without surgical interference.

Toothache

45.   There are several tens of cases in which toothache has
been relieved or completely removed in only one or

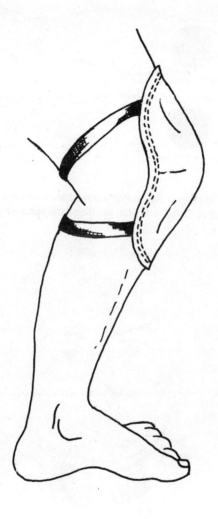

Kneet Belt: For pain and swelling of either knee. Apply the Knee belt on the painful knee for half to one hour.

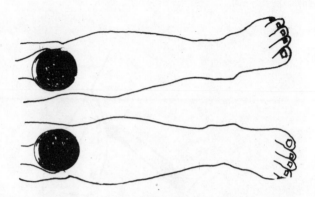

Treatment of Knees: North Pole on right knee and South Pole on left knee for treatment of Osteo Arthritis, swellings and stiffness or for other reasons.

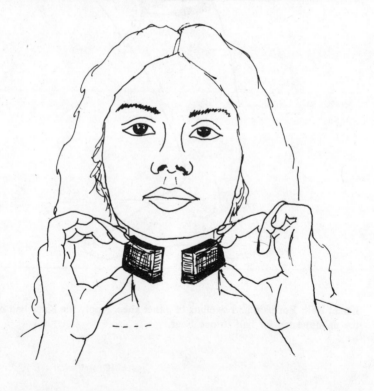

Throat Diseases: For irritation, cough and tonsilitis. Apply the Ceramic Magnets on both sides of the throat.

two sittings. The magnets were applied on the cheeks from outside in all those cases. The pains and swellings were wonderfully reduced.

The foregoing cases are only representative of the hundreds of cases of different diseases treated successfully with magnets. Some cases required surgery accordingly to the modern system of medicine but surgical operations were avoided by magnet-treatment and the patients were saved from the pains of knife interference.

Magnetotherapy has given most satisfactory results to the author in the treatment of eczema, spondylitis and toothache.

Views of an Indian Oncologist about cancer

Mr. Peshotan Mehta who has done research at the Swedish Hospital, St. Francis Hospital and the Fred Hutchinson Centre in the USA and has also attended courses at TIFR, Bombay, on "The Continuing Education in Oncology" as well as has done research in cancer feels that cancer is not a disease but merely an evolutionary process. He holds strong views against anti-cancer drugs and treatment such as irradiation which he feels damages cells and can kill patient faster than a cancer can. He is also of the opinion, which is shared by most of the Oncologists all over the world, that the more radical the extent of an operation, the lesser the survival rate among the patients.

The only rational cure for cancer, according to Peshotan, is Magnetotherapy. "Under normal healthy conditions all cells within an organism vibrate with a particular frequency. A cancerous cell has excessive frequency of a cell vibration. By applying magnetotherapy to it the frequency can be restored to normality." Research in this particular field is being carried out.

Dr. M.T. Santwani, Homoeopathician & Magnetotherapist, New Delhi.

1. *Paralysis*—My 65 years old mother-in-law had a sudden stroke of paralysis on the right side of her body. The paralised

parts were cold and there was a marked foot-drop. She was completely bed-ridden and had to be physically carried to toilet, etc. Two strong magnets were applied to both of her feet in the morning for 15 minutes and to her palms in the evening. After about three months of regular treatment, she was able to sit and move to the kitchen and bath-room alone with the aid of a stick.

2. *Rheumatism*—A 60 years old lady came to me for the treatment of rheumatism in both of her knees. She used to experience intense pain, specially during rainy season and. was unable to walk. She also complained of the increased salivation especially at night with the result that she had to get up and clean her mouth frequently at night. Two medium-sized magnets were applied to her feet for half-an-hour daily in the morning and twice a week to hands. After $2\frac{1}{2}$ months' treatment, she had astonishing relief in her pain and the water-brash also stopped.

3. *Pain in the Arm*—A 52 years old lady had sudden paroxysmal pain in her right arm. She also had a complaint of numbness in her left leg with the feeling as if drops of water were falling from her knee. High powered magnets No. 3 were applied to her right palm and left foot daily for half an hour. After two applications she felt 75% relief in the pain of her arm and after about one week, she was completely Okay.

4. *Headache*—A 54 years old lady was suffering from headache for the past 15 years. Often she also suffered from insomnia. She was advised to sleep with her head towards north and feet towards south which was in consonence with the terrestrial magnetism. In addition, she was advised to apply Ceramic magnets on her head twice daily. After 30 days of regular application, she reported great relief in her headache and she was able to sleep well.

5. *Inflammation and Bleeding of Gums*—A 35 years old person came to me for the treatment of inflammation, pain and bleeding of his gums. The examination revealed that his gums

had receded and he was suffering from acute gingivitis. Medium-sized magnets were applied to the gums on the outside. After about 20 minutes, the pain tapered off and was bearable. After regular treatment of 15 days, the inflammation, swelling and pain vanished. He was advised to use the magnets twice a week to prevent recurrence of the trouble. He was also advised to gargle with magnetised water which greatly relieved the bleeding condition of the gums.

6. *Pain in Shoulder*—A 65 years old man suffered from pain and stiffness of right shoulder. The pain extended to the elbow and to the fingers which were swollen when the patient came to me. He was not able to raise his hand without intense pain. He had been treated in American and all pathological/clinical tests had been carried out though without any result. Two strong magnets were applied to his shoulder and hand (North Pole to the shoulder and South Pole to the hand). After about a week the swelling of the elbow and fingers had completely gone and after three months of regular treatment, the pain and stiffness of the shoulder no more troubled him and he was able to raise his hand freely. He is alright for the past four years.

7. *Pain in Kidney Region*—Once I suddenly developed a terrible pain in my right kidney region around 5.30 in the morning. To my dismay, I found that I could not pass any urine except a few drops. The pain went on increasing. I immediately applied a strong magnet over the right kidney region and another one on the opposite side at the back. In addition, I started sipping magnetised water. After about 20 minutes, I passed a little urine and after about 40 minutes, I had profuse urination thereby relieving my pain and discomfort. The pain in the kidney region was dull and tolerable. I again applied the magnets in the same manner in the evening and on the following day, which permanently cured me of the trouble.

8. *Tonsils*—A 14 years old school going girl had a complaint of chronic tonsillitis associated with intense headache, coryza and sneezing. Two Ceramic magnets were applied on

the region of tonsils from outside which greatly relieved her pain in the tonsils and headache. After about two months of regular treatment, she was relieved of her troubles. It has been more than four years now and she has so far not developed the old trouble.

9. *Pain in the Leg*—A 9 years old girl had intense pain in her right leg. She could not sit or walk properly and the pain usually made her stoop. The pain was worse pressing. Medium-sized magnets were applied to her leg and foot. After about two sittings, she was relieved of her pain.

10. *Leucoderma*—A 13 years old girl is presently under my treatment for leucoderma. She has white patches all over the body, prominently on the legs, arms and temples. Two strong magnets are being applied once to her feet for 15 minutes in the morning and once to her palm for 15 minutes in the evening. After about a month of treatment, she reported that her patches were turning pinkish and that some of the light-coloured patches had become skin-coloured. Presently, most of her white patches on the feet, legs, hands and temples have become skin-coloured. She is continuing the treatment.

11. *Sciatica*—A 35 years old lady was suddenly seized with an intense pain in her left leg starting from the hip joint to the knees, after she got wet in a sudden down-pour. She took treatment from the Government Dispensary and Allopathic Doctors residing nearby her house but without any relief in her condition. Immediately after she approached me for the treatment, I applied strong magnets (North Pole) over the hip joint and the South Pole at the terminal portion of the pain *i.e.* knee. After about half-an-hour treatment, the intensity of her pain reduced and she was able to move. Another sitting was advised after 12 hours, After two days of applications, her pain stopped completely and has not recurred for the past one year.

Dr. A.C. Gupta, B. Sc., DHMS (Delhi) Nehru Homoeo-pathic Medical College and Hospital, Defence Colony, New Delhi.

1. *Cervical Spondylosis*—A middle aged lady consulted me for pains in the neck and shoulders extending to the arms. The

pain was more on the left side. The radiological examination showed disc degeneration (4th & 5th C.V.). Cervical traction and diathermy were of no avail. She came for homoeopathic treatment but I advised her to take magnetotherapy treatment. She was told to apply N-pole at the back of the neck (on the spine) and S-pole under the palm of the left hand. She reported full relief after 3 weeks. The pain has not recurred thereafter for 3 months.

2. *Chronic Tonsillitis*—A young girl of 12 years was advised operation for chronic tonsillitis. She had taken allopathic and homoeopathic treatment. The homoeopathic treatment relieved her symptoms but the enlargement of tonsils persisted. After one month of regular application of Ceramic magnets daily for 10 minutes, the size of the tonsils reduced by 75%.

3. *Enlargement of Prostate*—A middle aged patient was suffering from hypertrophy of prostate. He was admitted in a famous hospital in Delhi, with acute retention of urine. He was catheterized which afforded no relief. His son came to me for Homoeo treatment. I advised him to get the patient discharged from the hospital so that Homoeo treatment could be started. The patient was not discharged as he required constant catheterisation. When I was again approached to help him, I suggested that the patient may be given 2 oz of magnetized water every hour. It promptly cleared the retention of urine and the patient was discharged from the hospital within 2 days.

4. *Insect Bite*—My mother suffered from insect-bite with profuse swelling and agonizing pain around right eye. I gave Apis and Ledum (the usual homoeopathic remedies for Insect-Bites) but they provided only slight relief. Then I applied S. pole on the affected part for 5 minutes. The result was astonishing. Within two such applications on the same day the swelling and the pain reduced considerably. Application of magnet on further two days resulted in complete cure.

5. *Painful Abscess*—A 40 years old lady was under treatment in a hospital for traumatic paraplegia. One day she

developed pain and swelling in the left knee with fever. It was diagnosed as an abscess by the doctors of the Medical Institute. Allopathic and homoeopathic treatment failed to relieve this sudden development. After suffering for about 3 weeks, she applied magnets twice daily for ten minutes, below the soles of the feet. Within ten days, her swelling and pain disappeared. In addition to this, her stiffness of knees (an old symptom) was much relieved and she walked the whole length of the verandah twice with the help of callipers. She started feeling strength in legs and could extend her legs easily which she could not do earlier.

The application of magnets was accompanied by some burning tingling sensation and certain eruptions on the feet and lower abdomen which disappeared after few days.

Dr. M.C. Verma, D.H.M.S., W.Z. 6-B, Naraina, New Delhi-110028. Ex. Hony. House Physician, Nehru Homoeopathic Medical College & Hospital, Defence Colony, New Delhi, Consultant Homoeopathic Physician, Member : Homoeopathic Medical Association, Magnetotherapist and Chromotherapist.

1. My Grand Mother had a fracture of wrist-joint. She was under treatment at A.I.I.M.S. in Ortho-Physiotherapy Deptt., but the pain persisted. A Haemotoma developed over the wrist-joint. She took magnetic treatment for one month with North pole over the wrist-joint and South pole below the wrist-joint. After one month, the pain vanished altogether. To my greater surprise, the Haemotoma also disappeared. This created a tremendous confidence in me in magnetic treatment.

2. Mrs. Shashi Deep aged, 25 years was suffering from Cervical Spondylitis for the last three years. The pain started from the first thoracic region and reflected over the whole of the left hand. I applied North pole over the first thoracic region and South pole over the palm of the left hand for 15 minutes daily for about 45 days. There was a ring-worm over the neck. After magnetic treatment, to my greater surprise, not only the pain but also the ring-worm was cured.

3. Randhir Singh, a child of 6 years was suffering from Chorea and weakness of the lower extremities for the last 5 years. His hands trembled while writing or doing anything. Inspite of two years' treatment at Kalawati Saran Hospital, there was no improvement in the condition of the child.

By chance, his father consulted me and I took the child under my magnetic treatment. He applied magnets one day on the lower extremities and the next day under the palms. This treatment showed very slow progress but after one year's regular treatment the weakness of the lower extremities recovered the child's Chorea and showed excellent progress. Even his hands did not tremble at all. This was really a wonderful recovery in this case.

4. Pt. Bodh Raj Vashishtha was a victim of Migraine for the last 3-4 years. He had regular severe attacks of headache, twice or thrice a week. At last he stopped all other treatments and started magnetic treatment under my guidance. I applied North pole over his right side and South pole over his left side on the frontal region. After regular treatment of 4 months daily for 5 to 8 minutes, the patient completely recovered from the migraine trouble and he enjoyed perfect health.

5. I have treated many cases of displaced abdominal Aorta by placing South pole only over the umbilical region daily for 15 minutes. Satisfactory results are obtained even in 3 to 5 days.

In case of toothache also, application of South pole over the affected part gives a good response.

Dr A.K. Gupta, D.H.M.S., M.I.H.L. (Geneva) Homoeo-pathic Physician & Magnetotherapist, New Delhi.

Cervical Spondylitis

1. Shri D.P. Grover (53 years), an engineer in D.E.S.U., was suffering from stiffness and pain in the neck with headache and occasionally vertigo also. His case has been diagnosed as of cervical spondylitis. He had complaints for the last 6 years.

Nothing could give him the desired relief and after getting fed up from every where he started taking Magnetotherapy and to his utter surprise on the 23rd day of the treatment, he started feeling that the regularity of the pain had gone and the intensity of the pain had also been reduced tremendously. After continuing the treatment for 4 months, he never had the pains and stiffness again.

Frozen Shoulder

2. Mrs. Pushpa Dutta (53 years) was suffering from shoulder pains which used to radiate up to the arms with persisting stiffness and occasional numbness. Her case was diagnosed as of frozen shoulder. Having taken various treatments for pretty long, she could not be cured. As long as she took the medicines, she felt better but the moment she withdrew the medicines, pains again came up. After having the magnetic treatment for about a month or so, she never had the pains again.

Osteo-Arthritis

3. Shri Baldevraj (68 years) a retired army man was suffering from pains in both of his knees with swelling and stiffness and there were cracking sounds also while walking. He was suffering from these complaints for the last 12/13 years. His case was diagnosed as of Osteo-Arthritis. Winters and rainy seasons were the most troublesome parts of the year for him because his complaints used to become worse during that period. After taking every possible measure, he could not get relief. At last he started magnetic treatment half-heartedly and, to his utter surprise and wonder, after a month only, he found very encouraging progress and he started feeling better. On taking this treatment for another 3/4 months, he was perfectly all right and free from his annoying pains. And in winter I came to know that he had gone to Simla to see his son and daughter-in-law and from there he wrote me that after 12 to 13 years, he is enjoying the first snowfall again.

Progressive Muscular Dystrophy

4. Mrs. Chabbra (43 years) was suffering from 'Progressive

Muscular Dystrophy' of hands and legs for the last so many years. Her hands and legs used to remain icy cold even in summers. They were losing strength day by day and the rate of deterioration was very high. Inspite of the best available treatment, she didn't find any relief. Then she started the magnetic treatment and after about 2½ months, she started feeling heat in her hands and feet and they started remaining warm (at body temperature) throughout the day. In the 5th month of her treatment she started getting some strength also and now she could hold the things in her hands which used to fall down otherwise.

Post-Infection Polyneuritis

5. Master Jagjeet Singh (12 years), the only son of his parents, had hyperpyrexia (high fever) at the age of 8 years. He was given some injection by an Allopathic doctor. Fever came down immediately with profuse sweating all over the body, but the child couldn't speak, couldn't move his body. He was unconscious. He was taken to the Irwin Hospital and on the 3rd day of his admission he regained consciousness but with the effect that his left hand and right leg lost the muscular power and he could not use them. He could not open his left hand without putting pressure on the Metacarpophalangeal joints and he could not get up without taking any support. He could not put pressure on his right leg and hence could not stand straight and his normal gait changed. After taking the magneto-therapy continuously for 8 months, he started opening his hand without putting any pressure on the Metacarpophalangeal joints. At times he could get up without taking any support. His treatment is still continuing, of course he is taking Homoeopathic medicines also. Definitely, magnetic treatment has helped in his rapid progress.

Rheumatism with Wandering Pains

6. Mrs. Vimal Kumari (28 years), a teacher in a Govt. School, was suffering from persisting headache, pain in the neck, pain in elbows with swelling on the arms and legs. These complaints she used to get very often. She tried the neck

collar also for a few months but without any relief. She took short wave diathermy also. Then she came to know about the magnetic treatment. She took this treatment for about 4 months. After that, she never had the complaints again and she was free from the various pains. The first day when she came to the clinic, she could not get up from the sofa and was about to weep because of severe pains and now she climbs the stairs with smiling face.

Stiff Neck

7. Mrs. Manju Dhankani (31 years) had a very strange but an interesting story to tell about having the complaint of the stiffness in her neck. In fact her friend was suffering from the Cervical Spondylitis and her intimacy with that friend was very deep. So she started remaining mentally tense. This mental tension became the cause of the persisting stiffness of her own neck. She got her X-Ray of the spine done but it did not reveal anything abnormal, whereas still she was complaining of the stiffness. With the use of the North pole magnetic energy for about 12 days, she was free from that wretched stiffness for ever.

Swollen Foot

8. Miss Yashodhara (20 years), a candidate sitting for the I.P.S. competition had a swelling on the dorsum of her right foot for the last 8 months. Swelling was variable in nature, sometimes puffness became so marked and at times it used to disappear almost completely. She found this swelling when she was putting off her fleet shoes after playing badminton. At that time the swelling was so marked that she had to cut down the shoe to put it off. By taking magnetic treatment for about 1½ months, she became free from the swelling, which was painless throughout.

Shri **G.R. Chaurasia**, Naturopath; Magnetotherapist and Osteopath, 36, Naiwala, H. No. 1678, Karol Bagh, Arya Samaj Road, New Delhi-110005.

I have magnetised different types of vegetable oils and ointments. These oils/ointments are used in different types of diseases before I apply the magnets. Magnets inject the oils into the body to cure the diseases. With the help of these, the disease can be cured in shorter time, after the case is well-diagnosed. The following are a few cases treated by me :

1. Dr. Grover's father from Nizamuddin, New Delhi, was admitted in Willingdon Hospital for Hernia operation. After the operation, his urine was stopped. When the hospital doctor was about to do another operation, Dr. Grover came to me, took my magnetised water and applied the small magnets near the testicles, as suggested to him. Urine started coming out. I gave this treatment for 3 minutes after every 2 hours. The patient was cured of the trouble and no operation took place. The doctor was also surprised.

2. Shri Madan Gopal, Nagpur who was suffering from swollen prostate gland and swelling of his feet and hands, had fever. He was cured with the application of magnetised oil and magnetic treatment within 7 days.

3. Smt. Ram Piari, R.K. Puram, New Delhi, lost her appetite completely and had fever, swelling of feet, water from the body completely exhausted and vomiting could not be stopped. All these complaints were removed by my applying different types of metallic magnets and other treatment with the help of magnets. She was saved when doctors had lost their hope about her survival.

4. Mr. Parvinder Singh, Gautam Nagar, New Delhi, who was suffering from tonsils, was advised to undergo operation. As there was time, some body suggested magnetic treatment. He left the operation theatre and came to me. He was not registered with me earlier, but the case was taken up. Under my treatment with magnets he was cured without operation and has no complaints now.

5. Mrs. Y. Lakshmi from Nalgonda Distt., Andhra Pradesh, was suffering from glands, swelling in the chest and stone particles in one of the breasts, headache, blood clotting, veins swelling, leg pain, stomach trouble, etc. She was cured of all these

ailments with the help of different types of magnets and magnetised water. Ointments were injected through different parts of
her body to set right her spine with the help of magnets.

6.   Master Deepu, 9 years, Delhi, was not able to speak
even a single word. He was given the magnetic treatment, magnetised water, magnetic ointment and magnetised oil. He has
since started speaking and can speak well now. Defects from the
neck-gland were removed through magnetic treatment.

7.   Miss Poonam was suffering from some defect in the
spine, general weakness, pain in legs, fever, and her chest bone
was elevated. Her liver was not functioning well and she also
had gastric trouble, constipation, tonsils, infection in urine.
These complaints were removed with the help of magnetised
oil and water and application of North pole and South pole on
the chest.

With my technique, this therapy has been found to be very
effective in many other cases also where surgical treatment is
generally advised but is not needed and many diseases can be
cured if properly attended to.

I have been able to cure the following diseases with
magnets :

Bed-wetting, Breast diseases, Bronchitis, Cold, Cough and
Throat pain, Excess of weight (obesity), Hysteria, Mental fatigue,
Migraine, Painful menses, Pain in muscles, Pain in any part
of body, Primary stage of asthma, Pimples, Retention of
urine, Sleeplessness, Swelling of gall bladder and Swollen
prostate gland.

**Dr. P.K. Roy, M.B.B.S. Roy Pharmacy, 54, Central Road,
Calcutta-32.**

Orchitis

1.   Shri Dwineswar Singh, aged 15 years, of Jadavpur,
Calcutta-32, was suffering from pain and swelling in the left
testis which was tense and tender. I put magnets (South pole)

for half-an-hour twice a day locally from 27-11-1976 to 30-11-1976. Pain was relieved from second day. On 30th November, there was no pain and only slight swelling remained. He did not turn up since then.

2. Mr. S.K. Dutta Gupta aged 45 years of Calcutta-32, was suffering from low back pain due to early spondylosis of lumbar vertebrae. He was treated with magnets on both legs from 27-11-1976 to 13-1-1977 for 10 minutes daily and was completely cured.

3. Mr. Manisha Sen, aged 31 years, of Calcutta. I had to attend this case on an emergency call on 5-12-1976 at 5 P.M. Suddenly she got pain over her neck. On examination, I found that she could not open her mouth due to stiffness of sternomastoid muscle of left side. On 6-12-1976 Mrs. Sen entered my chamber with tears and with difficulty she managed to get on to my examination table. Her face was turned to the right side due to stiffness of the left sternomastoid muscle. I put magnets over the affected part. After half-an-hour, she opened her mouth with great relief. Treatment continued till 9-12-1976 with good results.

4. Mrs. Anu Roy, aged 31 of Calcutta-32, was suffering from weeping type of Eczema on her left palm for four months. Some ointments were given but she had only temporary relief. Magnet (N) was applied locally from 23-11-1976 to 6-12-1976 and she was cured.

5. Anandamay Bose, aged, 12 years S/o Mr. A.K. Bose, Calcutta-32, was suffering from Eczema on the dorsum of his left hand for two months. Magnetic treatment was started from 5-12-1976. There was no oozing of pus from 8-12-1976 and the condition of the skin improved from 16-12-1976.

6. Mrs. Manjusree Roy, aged 35, Calcutta-32, had Eczema over her right palm and back of right ear for a few months. She was under treatment of a Dermatologist. I asked her to continue quadedrum cream given to her by the previous doctor along with Magneto-therapy. Treatment was given on both palms

from 23-2-1977 to 4-3-1977. Her skin condition on both regions looked normal, after this treatment.

7. Mr. Sunil Dutta, aged 30 years, of Calcutta-32, was suffering from contact Dermatitis over dorsum of both feet for one month. Magnetotherapy was started from 17-3-1977. On 6-4-1977, the condition of the skin become healthy. However, I advised him to continue the treatment for a few days more.

8. Mr. Kausik Bose, aged 8 years, of Calcutta. It was a case of mumps. He complained of fever, pain and swelling of right side of neck on 20-3-1977. On examination, right parotid gland was found swollen, tense and tender. Magnetotherapy was started from that date on both palms and also locally. On 23-3-1977, left perotid gland also got involved. To my utter surprise I noticed on 24th March that no tenderness was there and all swelling was practically reduced to nil.

9. Mrs. Asha Das, aged 52, of Calcutta. She was complaining of pain of her both lower extremities after the operation of Gall Bladder in the year 1965. She could not sleep since then. I examined her on 9-2-1977 and put magnet under her feet for 10 minutes. After two weeks' treatment, she could sleep but she felt pain on the day when she did not put the magnets. She was on the treatment for 2 months. She did not take any medicine and this drugless treatment was quite satisfactory.

10. Miss Susmita Deb, aged 26, of Calcutta was suffering from pain on her legs for a few years. She used to take 3-4 analgesic tablets daily. I convinced her not to take such tablets. I put her on magnets and the treatment continued for two months. She was relieved of her ailments.

11. Mr. H.K. Mitra, aged 74, of East Calcutta, complained of pain in his lumbar region and right lower extremity and tremors of both hands. I examined him on 2.3.1977 and applied magnets on both hands and feet. After one month, tremors of hands disappeared and pain of lumbar region and lower extremity reduced to a great extent.

12. Shri Kunal Roy, aged 24, of Calcutta, M. Sc. Research student of Bose Institute, Calcutta. On 5.2.1973 Dry ice (Solid CO_2) was put over his right fore-arm by one of his research fellows for about 30 seconds. He came to me next day evening and was complaining of pain and swelling. I found there was induration and redness. I put Magnet (N) for half an hour. On 7.2.1977, 50% of his complaints were relieved. Treatment continued for about a week and he was completely cured. He did not take any medicine at all.

13. A gentleman aged about 38 years came to me on 30.11.1976 with the report of a noted surgeon of Calcutta. He had a history of undescended testicle on right side from birth. On examination right testicle was found absent and left testicle slightly enlarged, left spermatic cord thickened. Intra abdominal lump large size 10×7.5 cm firm, slightly moveable, side to side, not up and down, not tender. X-Ray, I.V.P. showed slight deviation of left ureter.

All the Surgeons suggested operation. I put him on magnet treatment under both feet and locally 'N' pole along with magnetised water. I examined him every month. After treatment of six months, the lump reduced. He did not complain of any thing untoward thereafter.

14. Shri R.M. Maitra, Calcutta-32, was suffering from pain and swelling of right big toe for a few days. I examined him on 31.7.1977. His blood sugar was normal and uric acid was 4.2 mg per cent. I gave him an oblong ceramic magnet and asked him to strap the magnet with North pole over the area. Pain was relieved from the next morning. He was completely cured within a week.

15. Mr. M. Ghosh, Calcutta, was suffering from Herpes over right side of chest and back. North pole of magnet was applied over the affected area from 24.7.1977 to 31.7.1977. He was cured.

Dr. K.P.V. Menon, Sreedevi Nivas, Palluruthy, Cochin-6. Registered Allopathic Medical Practitioner.

1. Mr. XX had his prostate gland removed in 1972 by

operation and since then his urine started flowing without any control. The poor fellow had to keep a turkish towel folded and to keep in his 'T' bandage all the time and change it every now and then. In 1973 he had another operation to correct it. He was sent to Bombay to have an expert opinion on his urinary system. They suggested another operation without any guarantee and so he refused and came back. He was highly disappointed and was passing his days till 2.3.1977. On hearing about my new magnetic system of treatment, he approached me and I applied the big set to his feet and the small one to the part of the abdomen. The flow steadily reduced and he was 80% cured. Magnetised water was also given to him during my treatment.

2. Mrs. A was suffering from Gall Stone and was to have an operation. Hearing about my free magnet treatment, she came to me to try her luck. Magnetised water was given freely to drink and the medium magnets were applied to both of her hands for 10 minutes, as she was a weak woman. She was wonderfully cured and on re-X-Ray the stone was found missing.

3. Mrs. X, aged 42, was suffering from Gall Bladder Stone. X-Ray showed the clear picture of the stone and operation was considered the only treatment. The poor woman was afraid of operation. She contacted me to try her luck. I gave her magnetised water and light magnets were applied directly to the affected area and high powered magnets on her hands and feet. for 10 minutes in the evening. After two months, X-Ray was clear and the patient was happy.

4. A Homoeopathic Doctor came to know of this wonder. He came to me with a Palpable Gall Stone without any pain or discomfort. I gave him 5 bottles of magnetised water to take home weekly and to everybody's surprise the stone could not be felt after one month. Only magnetised water was given in this case.

5. A Convent Teacher who was suffering from Asthma, T.B., Obesity and Blood Pressure came to me. I supplied her

a set of medium sized magnets with instructions to apply. After two months she came to my clinic and I could not recognise her. She was found to be in a picture of perfect health. She regained her health and is still continuing the treatment for 5 minutes daily.

6. A retired School Master had been suffering from acute Asthma and every morning he coughed in such a way as if he was going to die. He could not go out of his room for 6 years. To everybody's surprise, just after ten days' treatment, he became his old self and now he is a walking monument of my clinic.

7. A 18 years old boy was brought to me for Bed-wetting. The poor boy could not go to his relations or friends' house to spend a night because of the trouble. Magnets were applied to his bladder and also to his feet. He became normal after 15 days' treatment.

8. A boy of 16 years could not walk as his knees banged together and both of his legs were bent towards inside. He was treated by so many doctors who had failed. He was brought to me and by magnetic treatment he could run after two months.

9. A boy of 6 years was suffering from nervousness to strange places and people as well as from stammering. After local treatment to throat and to hands for 3 weeks, he was no more nervous and the stammering was also considerably reduced.

10. A boy of 17 years could not write without putting a heavy pad under the hand due to perspiration of the palm. The palm would always be wet due to excessive perspiration. He took my magnetic treatment and was cured in one month's time.

11. A 26 years old labourer could not go for work for the past eight years because of severe headache. He was given local treatment and magnetised water. He was cured of the headache and he started going for work by just five days' treatment.

12. An old lady with cataract was to go for operation but could not go as she had no money. She was treated with small set directly to both eyes for two weeks and considerable improvement could be noticed.

Cases treated by late Dr. M. Srinivasa Rao, 13/350, Achari Street, Nellore-524001.

Blepharitis

1. N. R. (Male) 60 years. Painful eye, lachrimation, angry red look. All other treatments failed. Relieved of the pain by the application of a pair of weak ceramic magnets for 15 minutes.

Cold, Cough, Headache and Lacrimation

2. G. K. (Male) 18 years. A small magnet with two poles applied on the temple, another between the two eye brows and another in the centre of the throat. Patient found relief after 2 weeks of treatment. Magnetised water was administered daily.

Constipation

3. M. H. 40 years (Female) suffers for the last 20 years. Magnetised water 2 ounces 3 times a day was administered. The patient got relief.

Dropsy

4. V. V. K., 72 years, Advocate (Male) was operated for Cirrhosis of liver in December, 1977 in Gandhi Hospital, Hyderabad. Later on he developed dropsy over his lower extremities and ascites in abdomen. All other methods of treatment were in vain. He was given magnetised water regularly twice a day. Application of magnets with Methods I and V and South pole over the region of the liver for a period of one month and a half (in June-July 1978). The dropsy and ascites disappeared and he is healthy now.

Diarrhoea and Fever

5. C. V. R. (Male) 23 years. Magnetised water every 2 hours controlled fever and diarrhoea. No other medicine was used.

Entero-colitis

6. M.A. (Female) 45 years. Severe Colicky pain in the abdomen, resulting in 6 or more motions every day for the last 6 years. Magnetised water and application of magnets over the abdomen gave relief after the treatment for a fortnight. Method of treatment—South pole on the liver and North pole on the left side of abdomen.

Hyperacidity

7. H. G. (Male) 33 years. Hyperacidity and flatulence for the last 6 years. General treatment in the morning with Methods I and V and 2 magnets over the abdomen in the evenings gave good relief after a fortnight of treatment. Magnetised water was also given.

Indigestion

8. M. S. N. (Male) 36 years suffering from chronic indigestion for over 2 decades. Medicines gave only temporary relief and there was recurrence on stopping the treatment. Daily administration of magnetised water gave him very good relief and general health and activity improved remarkably.

Insomnia

9. D.S.R. (Male) 68 years. Application of small magnet (South pole) between the two eye brows for 10 minutes on two successive days. He sleeps well without the application of magnet.

Obesity

10. K. K. M. (Male) 40 years. Dyspnoea on walking small distances, not able to squat on the floor. Methods I and V with South pole magnet on the back for two months. After one month's treatment, the measurement of waist has gone down by 12.5 cm. Now the patient is able to walk long distances easily. He is also able to squat on the floor with impunity. Magnetised water is being administered 4 times daily.

Pain in Arm

11. A lady had severe pain in the left arm suddenly and she could not move hand freely. Two poles of medium **Power**

magnets were applied, 4 times in a day as the case was acute. Within 24 hours, she was completely relieved of the pain and there was no recurrence.

Pain in Ears

12. K (Female) 60 years. Suffering for the last 20 years with severe pain and pricking sensation, four times in one hour in both ears. All types of treatment could not give any relief. After application of magnets with special treatment, there was a great improvement after one month.

Photophobia and Cataract

13. Mrs. R. 55 years. Due to old age there is extreme weakness and she is unable to move freely. Administration of magnetised water has created in her fresh energy. Special treatment for the eyes with South pole under the right hand and a small Ceramic magnet with North pole on eyes has improved her sight. She is more energetic and moves about with great activity.

Poliomyelitis

14. G (Female) 12 years. Left lower extremity more affected, suffering for the last 8 years. Application of magnets by Method V and South pole at the lumbar centre on the spine. The patient is very much improved after one and a half month's treatment causing wonder to the onlookers. Magnetised water was also administered.

15. V. L. (Female) 16 years. Severe affection of right lower extremity from her 5th year. Method V with North pole over the knee and South pole on the lumbar centre. 8 weeks' treatment was given. Now the patient was able to walk with greater ease.

Rheumatoid Arthritis

16. R. S. (Female) 60 years. Swelling of both the knees for the last two months. Magnetised water with application of

magnets by Method V and local application of South pole alternatively gave relief in one month, in June 1978.

Stammering

17. A boy aged 6 years. Stammering for the last 2 years. Crescent-shaped magnets applied on each side of the neck with Method I. Magnetised water was also administered.

Stiffness of Joints

18. M. K. R. 74 years, male, suffering from stiffness of joints of the lower extremities for the last 15 years. Magnetised water was administered. Application of magnets alternating Methods I and V for one month cured him marvellously, in June 1978.

A Huge Swelling on the Forehead due to Throw of a Missile

19. R (Female) 25 years. Suddenly a missile struck on the forehead and immediately there was a big swelling on the forehead with severe unbearable pain. South pole of a magnet for 10 minutes once in every 6 hours gave complete and good relief.

Weakness

20. A. S. M. (Male) 72 years. Due to age, the patient used to feel weak and unable to move out of the house. After administration of magnetised water and also application of magnets with Methods I and V, the patient felt energetic, moved out very well and was very active. Wonderfully, his eye sight was improved though he had cataract.

Besides the 20 case reports given above, it will be interesting to note down the following experiences of some patients sent by them in black and white. The joy of some other patients cannot be expressed in words :

(1) "I used to feel lethargic. And after few days of administration of magnetised water (wonder water) I am more energetic with vim and vigour".

(2) "I have got good appetite and my indigestion has disappeared".

(3) "An old person was astonished to say, "My grey hair has turned black—A marvellous change in me".

(4) "A magnetised water directly attacks the root of the disease, wherever it might be in the body without my knowledge, which I am not able to explain".

(5) Parents of the young children are very much pleased when the stammering of their children is reduced in a short time and when they see marked improvement to their astonishment in polio cases.

Dr. D.S. Murty, R.H.M.P., Viskhapattnam-530001 (A.P.).

1. Mr. S. (Male), aged 30—a port employee. Sciatica right side from $2\frac{1}{2}$ months. Pain was felt throughout the whole sciatica nerve and sudden clutches while walking. Allopathic medicines were used without relief. He came to me and I applied North pole to the hip and South pole to the foot. He was given magnetised water. He was completely cured in one month.

2. Mrs. P. (Female), aged 25—Rheumatic back pains, right leg and left hand pains for one month. She came to me and I applied North pole to the back and South pole to the hand and leg alternately along with magnetised water. She was cured completely in 10 days.

3. Mr. G. (Male), aged 35—Stiff neck and drawing pains in the left shoulder. He had to work hard for hours together. If he is strained, the stiffness and the pains increase. One year back he was admitted in the General Hospital under a specialist and contraction was applied. After 3 months he was discharged with some relief. He came to me. I applied both North and South pole to the neck on both sides and also under both hands for 15 minutes. He was given magnetised water. There was surprising relief after 3 months.

4. Mr. L. (Male), aged 40—Railway employee. Robust constitution. He is suffering from back pains for 3 months. He tried allopathy without any relief. He came to me and I applied North pole to the back and South pole to the hand alongwith magnetised water and Homoeopathic medicine. He was completely cured in one month.

5. Mr. G. (Male), aged 30—Post-operation case. Suffering from gastralgia for 2 years. He was operated by a specialist. On the next day, he was about to collapse with paralysis which the doctor declared was not due to operation. After one month he was discharged with gastric pain (for which the operation had been done) and with paralysis of left hand and left leg and vocal cord. He came to me then. I applied North pole and South pole to wounds and ceramic magnets to the throat on either side along with magnetised water and some Homoeopathic medicines. In 3 months' time he was relieved of the gastric pain from the leg. He was then able to walk and write and finally to talk as before the operation.

6. A boy, aged one year—Polio left leg 6 months back. He was not able to stand. He applied magnets throughout the leg from hip to foot daily for 5 minutes alongwith magnetised water. In 3 months, he was able to stand with the help of wall and cot etc. and walk.

7. Mrs. S. 60—Paralysis right hand and right leg three months back. As she was not able to move from her bed, she was given magnetised water and Homoeopathic medicine. In 6 months she was able to walk in her house.

8. Mrs. L. aged 60—The spine is hurt due to a fall some 4 years back. The last vertebrae of the spine is dislocated. The spine is curved and there is pain, when she moves. After eating or drinking, she is getting the water and the food into her mouth due to this bending position of the spine. She was applied North pole to the back where the vertebrae were dislocated and South pole to the hand alongwith

magnetised water.   In 3 months she was able to stand without any bend and the food and water was not coming into the mouth as before.

Dr. Neville S. Bengali, L.C.E.H. (Bom.) Aff. R.S.H. (Eng.) 7 "Firuz-Ara" 3rd Floor, Opp. Cooperage Band Stand, 160, Madame Cama Road, Bombay-400021.

Dr. Bengali has written a treatise titled "MAGNET-THERAPY"—Key to Good Health. He is a Homoeopath and a Magnetotherapist. He writes that Magnetotherapy can be used alongwith other modes of treatment. When done so, it certainly accelerates recovery and completes the cure. Besides furnishing general information about magnetic treatment, he has also given a number of cases treated with magnets. A few of these cases are briefly given below for the information of the readers of this book :

Paralysis and Sciatica

1.   Mrs. T. aged 78 years, was suffering from severe pains in the legs especially in the right knee and back. The pains were shooting down her legs with numbness. Her condition was diagnosed as Sciatica. She began to complain of numbness in her right hand also. Inspite of the treatment by specialists of modern medicine, her condition began to deteriorate. Finally, her legs were paralysed. After about 1½ months hospitalisation, the doctors said that her bones were "softened" and there was no chance of her recovery. She was then advised to consult Dr. Bengali for Magnetotherapy. At that time, she was suffering from severe pains, obstinate constipation and paralysis from waist downwards. She was given the first session of magnetotherapy on 31st March 1977 and she was given magnets to be used daily. Gradually her pains lessened. Her circulation improved and muscles became stronger. By the end of November 1977, she could sit up. Her arthritic pains also disappeared. All hopes had been given up on account of age but magnetotherapy brought out a truly miraculous recovery.

Retarded Child (Brain Damage)

2. Baba G.P. born on 28-8-1974 was a cesarean case and was put under observation immediately after birth. Doctors reported that the child's brain had not developed properly and this was confirmed by specialist's pathological investigations. In September 1974, the child was ill with cold and fever. Specialists again confirmed brain damage involving the speech centre. Consultation with eminent brain specialist of Madras was also of no avail. The child could not utter a single word in the beginning of 1976 and was unable to take a few steps. The brain specialists of Bombay also advised the parents not to undergo treatment with drugs, as it was of no use in his case. At the age of 2 years and 8 months the child had no speech and fell down even by taking two steps. His parents had heard that retarted children were helped by magnetotherapy. They started this treatment. Within one month, the child started talking and was steady on his feet. In October 1977, the child was talking and running about freely.

Rheumatoid Arthritis

3. Mrs. R.B.C. was suffering from chronic pains in her joints with stiffness. She also had severe pain in the nape of her neck extending down to her left arm. She was diagnosed to be suffering from Rheumatoid Arthritis and Cervical Spondylitis. She was taking some pain relievers and anti-inflammatory drugs and they gave her some relief.

Her pains increased in severity and the stiffness grew worse. Walking gave a lot of trouble. She started magnetotherapy on 29th October 1977 and began to drink magnetised water also. After a few days' treatment, she no longer needed any pain relievers. Her neck and arm pain had disappeared and she was cured of spondylitis. In December 1977, the Arthritic pains in her joints also disappeared alongwith stiffness und her movements became free and comfortable. She was 73 years of age and therefore she was pleasantly surprised to find that even at that age magnetotherapy could work so wonderfully.

Frozen Shoulder

4. Mrs. M., aged 48 years, complained of chronic pains in her right shoulder with stiffness. She was unable to raise her right arm above the level of the shoulder.

A powerful magnet was applied to her right shoulder on 1-6-1977. The South pole of a round magnet was applied to her right wrist. After one month's treatment, her condition was considerably better. Her movements were freer. On 10-8-1977 the pain and stiffness of her shoulder had disappeared completely. She could now move her right arm freely and comfortably.

Rheumatoid Arthritis (Surgical Condition)

5. Mrs. H.B., aged 44 years, was suffering from a persistent swelling of the right ankle with pain and restricted movement.

Her disease was diagnosed as Rheumatoid Arthritis with synovial thickening involving the right extra articular peroneal sheaths. X-Ray and specialists' opinion confirmed this. The surgeon advised operation of the ankle. On being afraid to undergo surgery, she wished to try magnetotherapy. The South pole of a round magnet was placed in her right heel for 15 minutes and a Cassetted magnet (with both the poles under her left heel). Such sessions were given twice a week. After four such sessions the swelling disappeared completely and the ankle movement was no longer restricted.

Facial Paralysis

6. Mr. M.P., aged 32 years, was suffering from heavy speech with paralysis of the facial muscles on the left side. He had developed these symptoms a fortnight back. He was advised to apply the South pole of a Ceramic magnet above the right ear for 15 minutes three times a day. He was also asked to place the magnet below the pillow at night with the South pole facing upwards. There was considerable improvement in his speech and the facial paralysis in about a week's time. After

a month the patient reported that his facial paralysis was completely cured and his speech had returned to normal.

Shri Gopal Chand Puri, 85-Kamal, 69-Walkeshwar Road, Bombay-400006.

Allergy

1. A man of 40 years suffered from some allergy 3 years ago and his face became black but the body remained fair as before The colour of face became as fair as the other body after 10 days' treatment. Methods used I & V. North pole water was also given.

Anaemia and Weakness

2. An elderly lady of 72 years, extremely anaemic and bedridden was cured in 15 days with magnetised water and Method No. 1. North pole was applied under right hand and South pole under left hand. She felt so energetic that she remarked : " I do not feel like lying down any more but what should I do." She has since started taking interest in religion and is extremely happy.

Arthritis

3. My wife was suffering from Arthritis for the last 20 years. Every time she had to limp for 5 to 10 minutes before walking. Only after the joints got warmed up, she could walk in a normal way. Now she has no pain in the knees and ankles and does not limp at all. Magnetised water and magnet treatment with Methods I & V were given to her for 3 months.

Constipation

4. A lady, aged 55 years, was in the habit of taking Laxatives (*e.g.* liquid paraffin or milk of magnesia) for the last 40 years. Constipation was her life-long ailment. She had developed several blemishes on her face and looked much older than her age. She was completely cured from her life-long ailment and looks bright and younger after just 30 days' treatment with magnetotherapy. Diagonal application of magnets. North pole under right hand and the South pole under left foot applied twice a day for 10 minutes each time. M.W. was

also given 4 hourly, 4 times a day, 50 ml. each time, for 30 days.

Dysentery-Diarrhoea

5. A girl of 30 years was suffering from severe attack of loose motions. She was passing 10 to 15 motions per day and lost 4 kg in 10 days. She tried allopathic treatment. Latest medicines were given but they were of no avail. Her father's death coincided with starting of Dysentery. She was brought to me in a dehydrated state. Actually she was being taken for hospitalisation and on the way they consulted me.

She was cured with Magnetotherapy. The response was immediate. I applied North pole on the belly, gave her North pole water every 2 hours and applied a small magnet South pole on the forehead in between the eyes. She was completely cured within 24 hours and the Dysentery did not recur.

(A small magnet South pole was applied on the forehead because I wanted to cover the nervous tension which was caused by the death of her father which in turn might have caused Dysentery).

Eczema

6. Colloid Lumpy, knotty, sticky knot, size of car head-light bulb. An old man of 66 years was suffering from this disease since 5 years on the chest near the shoulder. The itching was so severe that he could not bear it. He used to take strong sedatives to temporarily overcome the unbearable itching and catch up a few hours of sleep. It was weeping Eczema and his life was a real hell. He was completely cured with Magnetotherapy in 15 days. North pole was applied on the weeping knot twice a day for 15 minutes each time. North pole water given 4 hourly 50 ml. each time.

7. Another case of weepings Eczema. The patient was 40 years old and was suffering from this disease for $4\frac{1}{2}$ years. His both legs were affected up to the knees. It was difficult for him to put on pants because lower legs were inflamed and pain-ful. The very touch of cloth would aggravate his trouble. He

felt miserable as he could not bear it any more. As a result of this horrible disease he became unsocial. With Magnetotherapy he is not only completely cured, even the spots on his legs have disappeared. Duration of treatment 15 days. North pole water given. Applied magnets under the feet (Method V).

Knee Joint

8. A 95 years old man could not stand or walk. He was bedridden for more than 10 years. After treatment for 3 months now he can stand and walk. Two South pole magnets were kept with adhesive tape, one on each knee continously for 3 months. The adhesive tape was changed whenever it became dirty.

Morning Cold

9. A young man of 20 years was suffering from endless sneezing in the morning. His trouble was more than 5 years old. He was terribly sick. His morning cold and sneezing would start as soon he got up and lasted up to 1-2 0' clock in the afternoon. He had tried all sorts of treatments for several years but got no relief. He had also developed shortness of breath. He was completely cured in 15 days with the drugless healing method of Magnetotherapy. Treatment given Method No. 1, 10 minutes, Method No. V, 10 minutes. Alongwith Method No. V., 2 small magnets were used on both the sides of his nose. North pole on right nostril and South pole on left nostril for 5 minutes. North pole magnet was also applied on his forehead between the eye brows for 5 minutes everyday.

Multiple Troubles

10. A lady, aged 42 was suffering from several troubles simultaneously *e.g.* (*i*) Stomach ulcers, (*ii*) Infection in right ear with pus oozing out all the time, (*iii*) Killing pain in the head which made her life miserable, (*iv*) Sometimes feeling of collapsing in the kitchen while cooking, (*v*) Consequently she had become uninterested in life. All her troubles were 5 years old. She did not get any relief from any of the recognised treatment and had started feeling that she had reached a point of no return. When Magnetotherapy was suggested to her, she

laughed at the idea because she had never heard of it. Somehow she made up her mind to try it also and started the treatment. She started recovering from the 1st day and was completely cured of her ailments in 3 months. Necklace made of magnets was worn by her all the time for three months. North pole was applied on the stomach and under the ear. North pole water was given to drink. Magnets were applied under the hands as per Method No. 1. This case was treated in 1976 and she stands quite cured since then. She now lives a normal healthy life without any ailment.

Night Cramps

11. A boy, aged six years used to have severe pain in both the feet since birth. Several treatments of latest type were given but all in vain. The child would get up at night and complain of pain in the feet. With allopathic sedatives or pain killers, he would be put to sleep. This ailment was naturally a constant worry to his parents. In allopathy, the disease was termed as 'Night Cramps' and there was no cure for it. It was said that the pain would go when the child grows up. 'There was no remedy known to the science of modern medicine for this disease' as the parents were told.

The body responded to the very first application. Four strong magnets were used, 2 under the feet and 2 over the feet. Each foot having both North pole and South pole. Magnetised water was also given. The treatment was continued for 10 days only and the child was cured of the so-called incurable disease.

Rheumatism

12. A lady 30 years old was suffering from pain in each and every joint of her body for 8 years. She wanted to commit suicide. Her husband was at his nerves end and was a very unhappy man. She suffered all this at the time of delivery and her son was very slow in everything, weeping 4/5 hours during the day and about 2 hours at night. The boy learned to sit at the age of 4 and started speaking at 5 and was slow in picking up everything. The mother has responded to Method I & V

and magnetised water and is cured. The boy is normal with only magnetised water and nervitone (Allopathic Nerve Tonic). He does not weep anymore. I had not even seen the boy. He came to see me 2 days ago and behaved like an intelligent child. I asked him his name. He promised to tell me his name on the condition that I tell him my name first. I readily told him, "My name is uncle Puri.". He laughed it away and said, "I will not tell you my name as you are befooling me. How can 'Puri' be a name. We eat Puris. Do not try to befool me. He did not tell his name. Can anyone say that the boy was retarded up to 15 days back. Now it is a very happy family and offers thanks to Magnetotherapy.

All the persons whose histories are given above are in perfect health and willing to confirm that they got cured with Magnetotherapy.

Dr. Satram Das Lilani, Powai Chowk, Ulhasnagar-3 (Distt. Thane), Maharashtra

Magnet is a master manifestation of the nature which has been gifted to the mankind. This has been amply proved through various processes. If a human body is cut centrally and vertically in two equal parts, both the parts consist of limbs imbibing different magnetic polar qualities of the same strength. The right side of the body is charged with North (positive) while the left side is brimming with South (negative) polar properties. Through this magnetic power, we have started treating a number of ailments and some of my personal experiences are given below ·

1. Chronic Backache—A Gujarati woman resident of Vile-Parle (Bombay) was suffering from chronic backache which was declared incurable after protracted treatment by many reputed doctors. She was treated by placing South pole on her back horizontally for 20 minutes twice daily. After 40 days of treatment she reported 90% relief and could move and walk about on her own while previously she was confined to bed.

2. Disturbed Sleep—My wife always experienced disturbed sleep. I placed South pole below her pillow for 3-4 nights continously. She has been getting sound sleep every night since then.

3. Nail in Foot—A nail pierced the foot of the domestic servant of my friend. The injured foot was swollen and the patient was experiencing piercing pain. I advised him to place North pole below his affected feet and within half-an-hour the swelling and pain was relieved. He was advised to repeat the treatment the next day, as a matter of precaution.

4. Pain after Extraction of Teeth—After extraction of one of his teeth, my friend was suffering from swollen gum and severe pains which did not respond to conventional treatment. On application of North pole over the affected part for a short duration the pain and swelling were cured.

5. Pain of Accident—An elderly person was hit from behind on his back by a lorry and was admitted in a hospital where his backache was unsuccessfully treated. When he approached me, I applied high powered South pole over the affected part of his back two-three times and the pain vanished within 12-15 minutes.

6. Pleurisy—An elderly lady who was suffering from pleurisy for a long time is being treated by North pole magnetised water which was given to her for drinking. She is feeling much better with this treatment.

7. Sexual Excesses—A man in his late forties who had indulged in sexual excesses had lost his vigour. He was treated with South pole for a short period. He has since regained his vigour and is blissfully cheerful.

Dr. S.C. Gupta, Homoeopath and Magnetotherapist, Sonepat (Haryana)

1. The neck of Km. Veena Malik, B.A. age 18 years was bent towards the left shoulder right from the beginning. She could not move her neck to any side. There was pain in her neck between both the shoulders. Many treatments were carried

out but without any result. Doctors were of the opinion that there was no treatment for it.

One magnet (NP) was applied to her right hand and another magnet (SP) was applied to her left hand for one month. In one month, the pain in her neck subsided and it could move to some extent. The treatment continued for 4 months. She was also given magnetised water to drink 3-4 times everyday. Now she is quite free from pain and can move her neck to her right as well as to her left.

Syphilis

2. Shri Suresh Verma, aged 28 years, had ring-worm and spots on whole skin with great itching and burning for the last 20 years which sometimes resulted even in slight bleeding. The position of his skin had become pitiable. Highpowered magnets were applied to his palms in the morning and to his feet in the evening for 10 minutes daily and magnetised water was given to him for drinking 3-4 times every day for two months. His ring-worm and patches became alright and the marks of patches are also becoming like other skin.

Eczema

3. Shri Jagdish Agarwal, aged about 44 years, had eczema in both of his feet for the last 10 years. It was discharging profusely in the beginning but later became dry. It used to be highly aggravated in summer and rainy seasons and the feet used to get swollen. There was great burning and as a result of great itching the skin had become very rough, fat and black. Magnets were applied to his feet and magnetised water was given for drinking for two months. Firstly, his right foot which was suffering badly improved and after sometime the left also became O.K.

Tumours

4. A lady of about 22 years had some tumour-like growth towards her left as well as right ears. The tumour of the left side was of a size of an egg, was hard like stone and was painful. Two high powered magnets were applied to her palms for

15 minutes and one small magnet was tied to the tumour near her left ear. She was also given magnetised water to drink. In one month, the tumour became soft and began to shrink and the pain vanished.

5. Shri Gupta, aged 45 years, had got vasectomy operation done under F.P. in 1968. During the last two years there was no excitement at all in his sexual nerves and he began to feel himself quite impotent. For his treatment magnets were applied below his soles for 10 months continuously and one small magnet (South pole) was tied near his testicles and the sexual organ. Now he gets excitement in his nerves as before and he feels quite satisfied and happy.

6. A lady of about 30 years had pain and swelling in her legs, feet, soles, heels and found it very difficult to walk about. She felt some pain all the time. High powered magnets were applied to her soles for 10 minutes and to her palms for 5 minutes. After 20 days the swelling was gone and the pain was lessened. She became alright in two months.

Shri Ram Bilas Shukla, Vikas Sahayak, Block Narsingpur, Distt. Narsingpur (M.P.).

1. I have personal experience that increase of the growth of cancer is stopped within one month by the use of North pole of the magnet.

2. My common experience is that the magnet removes the excess growth of the flesh on the body as was noticed in the following two cases :

(*a*) Shri Purshotam Dwivedi, aged 60 years, a famous Vaid himself, had two big warts on both the sides of his neck. Both the warts were destroyed by the use of magnets within one month.

(*b*) I had a big wart in my foot and the same was cured by the application of magnets without any trouble within one month.

3. I have tried magnets on scorpion bites in several cases.

The sting of the scorpion and the pain was removed within 35 minutes in all the cases.

4. I have applied magnets on toothache and headache also and found them to be very useful in these ailments too.

5. The magnets were tried in the following Eczema cases and they proved very successful :

(*a*) Thakur Badri Singh, retired Tehsildar, had very bad Eczema on the whole of his body. His age was 55 years. The magnets were applied for one month. The Ecezma was fully cured and the complexion of the skin also became natural.

6. Smt. R.K. Singh, aged 35 years, wife of a teacher, got an attack of facial paralysis and her mouth became turned to one side and could not be opened fully. The vision of the right eye was gone. She was treated with magnets and was kept on natural diet. The vision of the eye came back within two months. The position of the mouth was also corrected and no trace of paralysis was left.

7. Shri Paramjit Panwala, aged 35 years, had pain and swelling in his feet and felt difficulty in walking about. On my suggestion, he kept a big magnet under his seat below some cloth. The trouble was removed gradually in two months and thus his rheumatism was cured.

15

Clinical Reports From Foreign Countries

Reports from Japan, U.S.A., Russia, France etc.

In the last century, Helmholtz (1821—1894), the most distinguished scientist and professor of Philosophy, of Germany aptly remarked, "The disgrace of the nineteenth century is its ignorance of the subject of magnetism; will the twentieth bring knowledge ?"

It seems that the people of twentieth century have taken the challenge seriously and have made satisfactory efforts to fulfil the expectation of Helmholtz.

The required progress has been made in many advanced countries of the world, including India, and all of them have made great progress in this field.

We are concerned here only with that part of magnetism which is applied to relieve and cure the ailments of the suffering humanity. In this particular branch also, appreciable progress has been made in countries like Japan, USA, USSR etc.

Reports from some Companies of Japan

A small but progressive country like Japan has promoted several companies which develop, manufacture and offer for sale several magnetic products for treatment of human ailments.

There is a company named 'Kawasaki Electric Industry Co. Ltd., of Japan, manufacturing electromagnetic therapeutic apparatuses. Their special product is an Electromagnetic Magnetizer. This is a sort of an easy chair fitted with

6 electromagnets. One has to sit in the chair comfortably up to half an-hour daily for some days, for getting relief from most of the common diseases.

A similar electromagnetic healing machine has been developed in India also by Dr. Satram Das of Saraswati Clinic, Powai Chowk, Ulhasnagar-3, Bombay, with certain further improvements.

There is another company named 'Nakatamasihki Medical Industry Co. Ltd. at Tokyo, Japan, who makes Magnetic Body Belts. The belts contain 16 Ferrite magnets built in it and relieve waist pain and muscular pain, etc.

Another company named 'The Aimante Trading Company' of Tokyo, Japan, is manufacturing several magnetic products for treatment of different diseases of human beings. Their main products are Magnetic Health Bands and Magnetic Necklaces. The health bands have achieved remarkable success in the cure of 'Stiffness of Shoulders' and 'High Blood Pressure'. The magnetic necklaces have been especially designed to decorate ladies while keeping them fresh, youthful and healthy. They also make 'Magnetic Bedpads' for removing constipation, fatigue and stiffness. These 'Bedpads' are said to be particularly beneficial for ladies for preserving lasting health and vigour. The company has managed to get many experiments about their Magnetic Health Bands carried out by different agencies including some hospitals. Some information about these experiments is given below:

An abstract of Biomagnetic Symposium held in Japan shows that the Japanese Scientsts and Doctors have carried out many laboratory experiments and have found that the relation-ship between magnetism and living bodies is of great interest and importance. Consequently, they have introduced magnetic treatment in hospitals utilising permanent magnets.

A report of the Tabata National Railway Hospital, Japan, has shown that the Magnetic Bands were used on patients visiting the hospitals at Chiba, Omiya, Shinjyoku. Tabata in

Japan and considerable effects on stiff shoulders and high blood pressure as the chief complaints of these patients have been confirmed. In most of the cases treated with Magnetic Bands, the complaints of stiff shoulders were relieved in periods ranging from 3 to 15 days and the high blood pressure from 7 to 90 days.

The abstract of the symposium shows that experiments were made with 42 patients suffering from stiffness of shoulders with or without other diseases. The report claims that the bands were found effective in 41 cases out of 42 and that many patients begain getting better within a week. The health bands were also tried on patients of high blood pressure. Thiry-four cases of various kinds of high blood pressure (simple, essential and pernicious) with or without other diseases, were tried with bands. Out of the 34 cases, the bands proved effective in 20 cases, non-effective in 8 cases and 6 cases remained undecided. In most of the cases in which the bands proved effective, the benefit was noted within a week or two and the blood pressure came down by about 20 mm in this period.

Reports from the United States of America

The United States of America have also made much progress in the field of application of magnetism for the benefit of the living beings. A number of doctors, institutes and laboratories have done appreciable work in conducting researches in this field. The names of some such doctors and institutions are given below, with the results obtained by them quoted in brief :

(1) Dr. Albert Roy Davis, the Director of Albert Roy Research Laboratory, U.S.A., has confirmed that he has arrested all forms of cancers, reduced tumors and controlled infections with the help of Biomagnetics. He writes that as a result of his research with animals, he has added to the years of normal life of the animals.

(2) Dr. Howard D. Stangle of New York believes magnetism to be a true science. He writes that it is all along

an admitted line that the magnet has hidden powers and that something of it has become known and been made use of from time to time. He observes that magnetism is among the truest things in life on earth and this view seems to have been shared by most eminent men of science—not merely of the West, but around the globe. He suggests that it is a subject that should excite universal interest.

(3) Dr. K. E. Maclean of New York city has been using strong magnetic fields in the treatment of advanced cases of cancer and the results are reported to be remarkable.

(4) Dr. M.F. Barnothy of the University of Illinois, U.S.A. and Dr. J.M. Barnothy of Biomagnetic Research Foundation, Evanston, Illinois, have found that bacterias change their positions relative to the magnetic field. Dr M.F. Barnothy hopes that magnetic fields will in due time develop into a powerful new analytic and therapeutic tool of medicine.

(5) Dr. Robert O. Becker, Professor of Orthopaedic Surgery, State University of New York, states that there would appear to be little doubt that some interaction exists between the function of the Central Nervous System and external magnetic fields.

Some cases treated by Doctors in America are given below :

Cases treated by Dr. Howard D. Stangle of New York

(1) *Heart Condition.* A man in late fifties suffered periodical attacks of violent nature seemingly pointing to "heart condition". His heart, however, seemed sound and it was thought that he might have got incipient cancer. He was advised to wear the North pole of a magnet next to his bare skin of the hip at a sore spot. The patient said that relief was felt within 2 hours of his wearing the magnet. He wore the magnet for several hours daily for several months. The heart condition

disappeared, pain lessened, digestion corrected itself and there was no need to avoid stairs.

(2) *Prostate Gland Enlargement.* A man in his late sixties suffered from an enlarged prostate gland. During the flare-ups, the pain was intense, business activities were suspended and there was little rest and sleep. Surgery was advised, but the man declined. He, however, agreed to wear a magnet. He wore one for several months. He did not get the old condition nor lost a day in business on account of his illness.

Experiences of late Dr. Albert Roy Davis, (Head of Department of Science, Florida, America).

(1) One day Dr. Davis found that his right foot and leg were not as tired nor did they ache as did his left foot and leg. He found that this was the result of his standing on his legs and feet next to a 1500-gauss magnet for about two hours, during an experiment on mice.

(2) So he undertook to strap a small magnet on his lower legs next to his feet. "No more tired legs or feet". A lesser force field acted to give his legs and feet just proper stimulation.

(3) He noticed that if after an accident or some damages to his person, he placed a magnet on the affected part, all pain would leave in 15-30 minutes.

(4) Dr. Davis once developed a bad painful toothache. He picked up a 300-500 gauss magnet and held it against his face next to the paining tooth. In 15 minutes, the pain lessened. He took a small magnet and placed it inside his mouth, between the inner cheek and the sore tooth. In four hours, there was no pain, nor it returned afterwards.

(5) He thought that a belt of small magnets around his waist would place him in a circular magnetic field. He obtained powdered magnetic iron and imbedded those

magnetic particles in a plastic strip. The gauss strength was reduced to 12 gauss per cm. He wore it one hour a day and found great improvement in his feelings and his health improved thereby.

(6) In an accidental explosion in his laboratory, his face, eyes, hair, ears and cheeks were covered with burning acid. The pain, partial loss of sight, burns, swellings of face and head were all unbearable. He applied a 2000-gauss magnet. In less than one hour, the pain and burning were reduced to about half its intensity. After the second day, there was no pain at all, and in 12 days all signs of acid burns disappeared and no scars were left.

Reports from Russia

The magnetic power is being used in Russia in different ways.

The magazine 'Soviet Land' No. 20 of October 1970, shows that magnetised water is being used in clinics there. In a Leningrad Clinic, patients suffering from stones in the kidneys and gall bladder drank this water and it held to wash out the salts and stones from their organism.

The journal 'Soviet Woman' No. 8 of 1973 published a news item that a woman in Turkmania swallowed needle when she was biting off the thread. Dr. D. Shukorov tied a small magnet to a thread and got the patient to swallow it. Then he pulled out the magnet with the needle stuck to it.

Russians have recently come out with another noble idea relating to magnetic surgery for certain cases which defied effective surgery earlier. Dr. Leman who often performs operations for removal of foreign bodies from various human organs was puzzled over the problem of how to remove a foreign body from the respiratory tract with as little injury to the patient as possible. He finally decided to use the magnet's properties which are already known to the medical man. He designed a special instrument which could be introduced into the respiratory tract and bronchi—a tube of ferro-nickle steel.

A magnet was mounted above the operating table, and as the tube was lowered into the bronchi and came close to the metal item, the later stuck hard to it. The whole operation without any scalpel, forceps or blood-letting, took just a few minutes. With the initial success, Dr. Leman has now designed a set of apparatus and instruments for magnetic surgery. The electro-magnetic laboratory at the Institute of Metal Physics of the USSR Academy of Sciences, Ural Scientific Centre have now evolved magneto-metric installation which can remove almost any foreign metal body, without any damage to the patient's organism. Dr. Leman asserts that the magnet has become his faultless and efficient 'assistant' in operations not only on the respiratory tract, but on the esophagus, liver, duodenum, heart, etc.

There is a museum to display, in glazed show cases, various metal pellets, nails, coins, buttons, pins and needles, etc. which have been extracted from human bodies in the first City Hospital in Sverdlovsk (the Urals region) in Russia.

Reports from Italy

Prof. D. Gigante of the Institute of Rheumatology of Rome University made some clinical researches on the patients suffering from various kinds of Rheumatism and reported the result in 'Recentia Medica' of April 1966. Some extract's from his report are given below :

"Our observations concern 40 patients with various rheumatoid conditions at different stages. The results effected in the 40 patients show that one can without doubt affirm that the painful symptoms were influenced by the magnetism.

In 25 patients, the pain reduction varied from moderate to total.

At the level of articular and periarticular tissues, in which acute inflammation was present, the beneficial effect was particularly evident.

On the whole, the patients felt more tranquil, became more mobile and increased their resistance to fatigue. During the experiments, no side effects occurred at all and no harmful intolerance or reaction appeared.

"In the clinical aspect, the longest wave produced by magnetiser showed the most excellent anti inflammatory effects, leading to subsidence of pain symptom".

Prof. A. Venerando, Commissioner of C.O.N.I., Institute Di Medicina Dello Sport, also carried out some clinical research on the patients suffering from various Traumatisms caused by sport playing, such as arthritis, arthralgia, pains and musculature and recovery from heavy fatigue. The details of the results have been reported in the Gazetta Internationale Di Medicina E Chirurgia of Rome for May 1966.

The author experimented on 86 cases of acute and chronic articular musculo-tendineal and enthesopathical lesions, seen in athletes, with magnetiser. The action of this therapy resulted in marked reduction of the muscular constructure and of the painful symptoms.

The treatments were carried out with one or two electromagnets, coupled according to the area. The use of pairs was suggested with the object of rendering the penetration of the electromagnetic lines of force better and more intensive. The most favourable result was obtained in the reduction of pain and local swellings.

The use of couples of magnets reported to in some of the above mentioned cases in Italy was in accordance with the use of pairs of magnets suggested in the methods of treatment recommended in Chapter 10 of this book.

Reports from Scandinavia

A report prepared by Dr. Christine Pickard speaks about several cases treated successfully by magnetotherapy. The cases related to gall stones, heart attacks, heart cramps, high blood pressure, kidney stones and rheumatic pain and many subsidiary symptoms associated therewith. Giving the details of all those cases will amount to repetition of the same course

of diseases and treatment. It will suffice to add that in some
of the cases reported, the results of the magnetic treatment were
very remarkable and appreciable.

Some other countries are also making researches and experiments with magnets, magnetic fields and magnetic apparatuses
and their results are bound to be encouraging and a step further
for the betterment of the sufferings of the human beings, in due
course of time.

Reports from France

Malignancy, which is afflicting human race without any
bias for creed, colour and sex, has drawn attention of the
medical men and scientists all over the world. Concerted efforts
are being put in to find out rational and simple cure for malignancy or cancer.

In recent years, an Italian electronicist working in France
has been experimenting on magnetic field for the cure of malignancy. He has shown that remission of malignancy can be
effected after treatment in an intense magnetic field generated
by the machine built by him. This corroborates the observations
of Dr. K.E. Maclean of New York that "cancer cannot exist
in a strong magnetic field".

Reports from Australia

Use of magnets in almost all branches of medicine and
surgery has inspired a number of dentists as well, for their
employment against toothache and decayed teeth and for holding
dentures in place. A new method of holding dentures with
mini-magnets has recently been developed by an Australian
dental surgeon. The dentician has used tiny magnets made by a
surgeon. The dentist has used tiny magnets made of an alloy
of cobalt and a rare metal namely, samarium, which are about
ten times stronger than normal magnets. The method has been
developed and perfected by Dr. Barry Gillinges of the Department of Prosthetic Dentistry at the University of Sydney. The
magnetic dentures used by him are coupled with smaller magnets
implanted in patient's teeth stumps.

Part VII

16

Magnetotherapy and Homoeopathy

Magnetotherapy closely allied to Homoeopathy

Magnetotherapy is closely allied to Homoeopathy and has its backing.

The founder and Master of Homoeopathy, Dr. Samuel Hahnemann, in his book "Organon of Medicine" has pointed out the aims which every physician should keep in mind. He has stated as follows :

Section I. "The physician's high and only mission is to restore the sick to health, to cure as it is termed"

Section II. "The highest ideal of cure is rapid, gentle and permanent restoration of the health or removal and annihilation of the disease in its whole extent, in the shortest, most reliable and most harmless way, on easily comprehensible principles."

It was with this idea in Hahnemann's mind that besides Homoeopathy, he sought for the truth in the effect of and the relief through other methods of treatment prevalent in his time. He studied all the systems prevailing then and has given his opinion about them in the new sections 286 to 293 of the sixth edition of the Organon of Medicine.

Dr. Hahnemann has stated in the new section 286 ibid that the dynamic force of mineral magnets, electricity and galvanising act no less powerfully than the Homoeopathic medicines. In section 288 he has observed that animal magnetism (or mesmerism) is a marvellous priceless gift of God to mankind and

221

in section 289 he has mentioned about the positive and negative mesmerism as well as about the positive and negative 'Passes'. In section 290, he has spoken about the utility of massages and in section 291 about the benefit of water and bath as remedial agents.

Hahnemann and Mesmer were Contemporaries

Dr. Samuel Hahnemann (1755—1843) and the pioneer of magnetism and mesmerism, F.A. Mesmer (1734—1815) were contemporaries. Hence Hahnemann knew many magical cures performed by Mesmer by his magnetic or mesmeric treatment and was naturally influenced by these cures. Hahnemann, therefore, made experiments with magnets for a long time. When he was fully convinced about the beneficial effects of magnets, he wrote strongly in favour of their use. An extract of the new section 287 of the sixth edition of the Organon is given below :

Section 287 : The powers of the magnet for healing purposes can be employed with more certainty
according to the positive effects detailed in
the Materia Medica Pura under North and
South pole of a powerful magnetic bar.
Though both poles are alike powerful, they
nevertheless oppose each other in the manner
of their respective action. The doses may be
modified by the length of time of contact
with one or the other pole, according as the
symptoms of either North or South pole are
indicated. As antidote to a too violent action,
the application of a plate of polished zinc will
suffice."

Dr. Hahnemann, in his great work "Materia Medica Pura, Volume II", has devoted 54 pages to the treatment through magnets and through the medicines prepared from the magnet. He has given detailed information about magnets including the method of their preparation and has devoted 448 pages to describing the symptoms covered by the medicines prepared from the three different properties of the magnet.

Observations of Dr. Hahnemann about Use of Magnets

Dr. Hahnemann has made, *inter alia*, the following observations regarding magnets and their use :

"A magnetic rod can quickly and permanently cure the most severe disease for which it is suitable medicine,* when it is brought near the body for but a short time, even though covered with some thick material (such as cloth, bladder, glass, etc. **)

Although each of the poles presents something peculiar in its power of altering the human health, yet each of them seems to produce alternating actions which resemble those of the opposite pole.

In order to effect a cure, the magnet must be applied in a much milder manner to enable it to act homoeopathically.

For this purpose, a magnetic rod which can lift a quarter of a pound at either pole is more than sufficiently powerful.

I have met with cases for which the contact of such a magnetic staff for only half a minute was an amply sufficient dose.

If the wrong pole has first been selected, the opposite pole should be applied.

A mild disposition, or a tendency to chilliness in the subject of treatment, directs the practitioner first to the North pole when he can only find the symptoms similar to those of the case in hand, under the general magnet symptoms.

---

* It may be noted that Dr. Hahnemann has called the Magnet "a suitable medicine" here. He has truly called it. so as Charak, a most renowned authority on Ayurvedic System of treatment has also said "That which restores health is the proper remedy, he who cures the patient is the best physician".

** "Cardboard, paper, rubber, stainless steel and wood" may also be added to the list.

The duration of action of a moderate dose of magnetic power is upwards of 10 days.

"When the magnet has been improperly selected, the resulting sufferings, which are sometimes very severe, will be permanently removed by laying the outspread hand on a pretty large zinc plate for half an hour."

Three Magnetic Medicines

Three separate medicines are prepared in Homoeopathy from the three different properties of the magnet, namely : (*i*) The whole magnet, (*ii*) The North Pole, and (*iii*) The South Pole.

The medicine prepared from the whole magnet, named Magnetis Poli Ambo. covers, 397 symptoms ; the medicine prepared from the North Pole, called Magnetis Polus Arcticus, covers 459 symptoms; and the medicine prepared from the South Pole, called Magnetis Polus Australis, covers 387 symptoms. Thus all the three medicines prepared from the magnet cover 1243 symptoms. Fifty symptoms out of them are printed in bold type in the Materia Medica Pura and are, therefore, important symptoms for the use of the magnetic remedies.

Hahnemann has stated that the symptoms occurred from various powerful magnets brought in contact with various sensitive individuals without distinction of the poles. They were observed in experiments conducted for half a year for the purpose of ascertaining the proper and most efficacious mode of stroking the steel with magnets, in which a horse-shoe magnet capable of lifting twelves pounds was held in the hands, which were in contact with both poles for an hour at a time.

Dr. H.C. Allen Writes a Great Deal about These Three Medicines.

Dr. H.C. Allen, M.D , a great and renowned homoeopath, has written much about the magnet and the magnetic medicines in his Materia Medica of the Nosodes (with provings of the X-Ray). He has devoted 48 pages to the description of the magnet, giving the original remarks of Dr. Hahnemann, and to the description of the three magnetic medicines.

Most of the symptoms described in Dr. Hahnemann's Materia Medica Pura have been noted in Allen's Materia Medica of Nosodes. More important of Hahnemann's symptoms have been side-lined in Allen's book with double lines and less important symptoms have been side-lined with one line. Ordinary symptoms have been printed without any side-lining.

Almost all the more important and less important symptoms included and side-lined in Allen's Materia Medica mentioned above have also been given in his "Key Notes and Characteristics with comparisons of some of the Leading Remedies" without side-lining any symptom. The 'Key Notes' also give other symptoms not side-lined in the Materia Medica. As the Key Notes contain much less number of symptoms than those given in Dr. Hahnemann's Materia Medica or Allen's Materia Medica of Nosodes, it can be safely assumed that all the symptoms printed in the Key Notes are selected symptoms and are, therefore, important and dependable ones. Mention of the three magnetic medicines is also found at two places in the Boericke's Pocket Manual of Homoeopathic Materia Medica as well as in other Materia Medicas. Thus it is clear that the treatment of diseases through magnets and magnetic medicines has been up-held and recommended by the masters of Homoeopathy.

It is not possible to give all the 1243 symptoms indicated in Hahnemann's Materia Medica Pura, Volume II, in this book, for obvious reasons. The most important fifty symptoms printed in bold type in that book are, however, given here for the information of the physicians and others who wish to use the magnetic medicines for relieving these symptoms.

Important symptoms of the medicine prepared from the whole magnet, named **Magnetis Poli Ambo**, printed in bold letters in the Materia Medica Pura, Volume II :

Page of MM	Sl. No, of Symptoms	Symptoms
1	2	3
66	30	Sweat on the face, without heat, in morning.
69	94	Hunger especially in the morning.
70	123	Very loud rattling and rumbling in the adbomen.
70	141	After the stool, violent haemorrhoidal pain in the anus, sore as from a wound and a constrictive sensation more in the rectum than anus.
71	145	Haemorrhoidal flux.
71	156	Nocturnal pollution.
71	160	Absence of sexual desire.
71	162	The prepuce is retracted behind the glans-penis and does not cover it at all, or only to a very small extent.
72	175	At night and at other times, a violent but short fit of dry cough, after which there comes a slight expectoration of ordinary tracheal mucus.
72	178	Mucus in the trachea, which is easily expelled by short cough in the evening and morning.

1	2	3
73	203	Pain in the sacral articulation in the morning in bed, when lying on the side, and by day during prolonged stooping forward.
74	229	Drawing from the head to the tips of the fingers.
79	345	Waking up at about 3 A.M. after some hours of dreamful slumber, then without thirst sensation of heat in the limbs, which he first wishes to have uncovered, afterwards carefully covered up.
79	348	In the morning, he lies asleep on his back, one open hand lies under his occiput, the other over his stomach, with the knees spread out, with snoring during inspiration, with half open mouth and low-talking in sleep; he dreams amorous subjects and seminal emissions (though none occurs) after working headache in the occiput, as after a pollution, tightness of chest and bruised pain of all the joints, which goes off after rising and moving the body, while a large quantity of catarrhal mucus is thrown up.

1	2	3
81	378	While at his work during the day, he talks aloud to himself, without knowing it (immediately).
81	392	Very much disposed to get angry and indulgent, and when he does get angry, he has headache of a sore description (immediately).
81	394	Irascibility.

Major Symptoms of the Medicine prepared from North Pole (Magnetis Polus Arcticus)

1	2	3
84	47	Stitches in the eyelids.
84	54	Twitching and drawing in the eyelids.
85	56	Drawing in the eyelids and lachrymation.
85	60	Itching in the eyelids.
85	62	In the morning on awakening in bed, painful dry feeling of the eyelids.
85	70	Coldness of the weak eye, as if a lump of ice lay in the orbit instead of the eye; when the coldness went off, a prolonged needle prick in the eye.
85	73	Restless motion of the eye.

1	2	3
88	149	Frequent eructation of nothing but air.
88	I65	Gurgling in the abdomen, as if much flatulence were incarcerated, which causes also a twisting about that mounts up into the scrobiculus cordis and occasions eructations.
89	183	Hard, large-sized, rare stool, passed with difficulty.
90	193	Dark urine.
90	203	Noctural pollution.
90	210	The catemania, which were expected, came on in 20 hours, increased in 24 hours beyond their usual quantity—(they had hitherto been too scanty)—and became healthy in amount, without any more accessory symptoms (consequently curative action).
91	240	Itching in the region of heart.
95	344	Trembling in the parts touching the magnet.
95	347	Cold sensation on the place of application.
96	365	Great drowsiness ; he must yawn.
96	386	About 2 A.M., half waking, with much inner consciousness, great wealth of thoughts

1	2	3
		and lively memory; he thinks of an important subject in the best form in a foreign language with which he was not very conversant; almost as if in a zoo, magnetic sleep-talking state, but when fully awake he cannot remember distinctly the subject of his thoughts.
97	391	At night collection of saliva in the mouth, so profuse that each time he wakes, the pillow is quite wet.
97	402	Chill, shivering.
97	407	Cold sweat on the hands and soles of feet.
99	438	Anxious, dejected, fainthearted, inconsolable, disposition that caused him to make self-reproaches.
99	442	Anxious scrupulosity.
99	453	Hasty-hurried.

Major Symptoms of the Medicine prepared from South Pole (Magneus Polus Australis)

1	2	3
101	38	Watery eyes occasionally.
101	41	A painful sore dryness of the eyelids, felt especially when moving them, chiefly in the evening and morning.

1	2	3
101	48	Defect of vision, objects appear dim, then also double.
103	85	Burning in the gullet.
107	207	In the arms, quick painful twitching downwards.
108	249	An aching tearing in the patellae.
109	273	Shooting in the soles.
111	320	Dreams of incendiary fires.
112	365	Warmth all over, especially in the back.

It will be better, if while administering the magnetic medicines for relieving the symptoms noted under them, the whole magnet or the particular pole of the magnet, as the case may be, is also applied to the affected part of the body, with a view to getting quicker relief.

Dr. Neville S. Bengali of Bombay has written in his book "Magnet-Therapy" as follows :

Dr. Hahnemman's concept was far ahead of his time, as very little was then known about the electro-magnetic nature of cellular activity and the importance of magnetism. However, today we know that every homoeopathic remedy is the electro-magnetic energy of that particular substance. The substance that is to be made into a homoeopathic remedy is repeatedly subjected to processes known as "trituration" or "sock succus sion", by which the atoms of the substance are split, releasing the electro-magnetic energy pertaining to that particular substance.

Homoeopathy is thus complimentary to magnet-therapy as homoeopathic remedies do not possess any chemical substance, but the dynamic (electro-magnetic) energy of that substance which is obtained by potentising, which produces magnetic fields of different strengths.

With increasing potencies the electro-magnetic frequencies of the drug substance increase.

"The lower potencies, that is from the 3rd to the 12th, correspond to the lower frequencies; the 30th and 200th to the medium; and 1000 and above to the highly penetrating higher frequencies. As the potencies increase, the remedy becomes more deep—acting and long-acting. This makes homoeopathy, like magnet-therapy, the treatment of choice in all chronic and long standing ailments".

It may be concluded from the above that while low-powered magnets may be applied in new and light diseases, chronic and severe cases require the application of high powered magnets and for longer periods to get good results.

17

Magnetotherapy and Acupuncture or Acupressure

Acupuncture Points can be Utilised for Magnetotherapy

Hitherto, we have dealt with the local and general application of magnets against various diseases. While the local treatment has been suggested for alleviating the localised pain and stiffness in a particular spot, the general treatment has been directed against the diseases in the whole organism.

The author fully appreciates the efficiency of the above mentioned methods, yet, in an era of growing science and technology, one cannot close one's eyes to more accurate methods of application, provided they are fully proven and promise a better cure.

This concept led the author to study and find out the possibility of utilization of various acupuncture points in magnetotherapy for treatment of various internal ailments.

Acupuncture is Ancient Chinese Art of Healing, which has since been adopted by Japan and by some Western countries like the United States of America and England. India also is taking to it now and several physicians have started practising it in this country.

Acu means needle and puncture means pricking. Hence Acupuncture means treatment of patients through the art of pricking or piercing needles on some special points on the body of the patients. In the practice of Acupuncture, a fine needle is pierced into the skin of the patient to the depth of a few millimetres and is withdrawn after a few minutes. The most important thing in the practice of acupuncture is to know which point is to be pierced in a particular disease.

233

The ancient Chinese made no distinction between arteries, veins, nerves, tendons or meridians. They were concerned with a system of forces in the body, which enables a man to move, to breathe, to think, etc. The main concept of Chinese was life energy called *Qi* (pronounced chee). The man's possession of life and all its activities are believed by them to be completely dependent upon this *Qi*. In Hindu terminology, the nearest equivalent to *Qi* is *Prana* ; in Theosophy and Anthroposophy, it is called Ether. The *Qi* is created in human body by breathing and eating.

Acupuncture Points

The acupuncturists believe that there are tender areas at certain points on the surface of the body in all diseases and these tender areas are the Acupuncture points.

In simple acupuncture diagnosis, the patient is examined from head to toe in order to find out all the tender points and to deduce the internal disease corresponding to them. It has been noticed that a disease of an internal organ produces pain, tenderness, hyperesthesia or hypoesthesia, etc. in some part of the skin. This can be varified experimentally.

There are several systems of treatment through acupuncture. In one system, the tender points are needled while in other forms the acupuncturists prick those points where no pain is felt at all or the points which are often remote from the seat of the disease, and sometimes on the opposite side of the body.

The Indian points of *Chakras* correspond to acupuncture points. The Mahaout prods special places on the body of his elephant, with a sharp stick, to elicit various responses from the animal. Several indigenous medical systems in different parts of the world seem to correspond to simple form of acupuncture. Some Arabs cauterise part of the ear with a red hot poker for treating Sciatica while some Bantu Healers of South Africa scratch small areas of skin and rub various herbs into them.

In Chinese literature, about one thousand acupuncture points have been described—these may be even more. The thousand or so acupuncture points may be divided into various categories, all points in each category having similar properties.

The acupuncture points that are near the site of symptoms often have a greater local effect, especially in painful conditions. Points that are far away, especially the important points below the knee and elbow, often have a greater systemic effect.

Various Ways of Stimulating the Points

There are various ways of stimulating the points, namely, electrical stimuli, magnetic oscillations, mechanical vibrations, injections, massages, etc., besides puncturing the points with needles. There are also different ways of practising acupuncture. The needles are made of several materials, namely: silver, alloys, stainless steel and even gold. The Chinese books describe about fifty different ways of inserting needles. The technique involves inserting needles 3 or 9 or 81 times, twisting the needle clockwise or anticlockwise, inserting the needle fast and taking it out slowly, inserting the needle in three stages and pulling it out in one, and in many other ways. The stimulus differs with the thickness of the depth of insertion, the up and down pushing of the needle, bluntness or sharpness of needle, leaving the needle in body for longer times and repeating the treatment at frequent intervals.

For a more serious study of Acupuncture, the reader is referred to a detailed treatise on the subject by Dr. Felix Mann.

Certain Clinical Cases

Dr. Mann cites innumerable clinical cases where simple acupuncture techniques helped obviate complicated conditions. One such instance is that of a patient who sprained her wrist and suffered from palpitation. Considering that the tender point on sprained wrist crossed the heart meridian, he treated the point near wrist and cured the lady of her palpitation.

In another case, where a lady patient had painful periods, the needle was applied on the inside of the knee on the liver meridian (as the meridian has an indirect course to reproductive organs).

Similar cases have been reported by the author in this book in his treatment through Magnetotherapy, where the treatment against weakness and heaviness of legs improved the menses of the patients (for detail, please see Chapter 13 under the cases treated by the author).

The Chinese describe the acupuncture points as being quite small—a matter of millimetres—but there are Western acupuncturists who do not subscribe to this view and believe that a stimulus anywhere in the appropriate determatome will work. Both of them may achieve equal results if the oriental's acupuncture point lies within the area of hypersensitivity of the occidental. This shows that the area around an acupuncture point absorbs the effect of stimulation and the central acupuncture points or the lines of meridians are like the lines of force around a magnet and postulate a magnetic theory.

Some doctors have tried to combine acupuncture with the principle of Western physiology, anatomy and medicine in general.

The idea of combining acupuncture with medicine in general seems to be far-fetched, but the view that the stimulation of the area near or around an acupuncture point will give good results appeals to reason.

As there are more than a thousand acupuncture points in the human body, the points must be quite small and each of them must be fixed in a very small space in the body. It is naturally difficult, therefore, to locate the exact points of acupuncture for piercing the needles. There are also great chances of wrong points being pricked as some of them are very closely placed.

Acupressure

Besides the use of needles, the practice of Acupressure, *i.e.*

Acupuncture without needles, is also gaining popularity on account of its simpler approach.

In his interesting and profusely illustrated book on Acupressure, Dr. J.V. Cerney of U.S.A. has recommended the use of pressure by one's finger-tips. According to him, different acupuncture points either need stimulation by light, soft and superficial pressure to tone up the tissues involved or they require sedation by deep and slow pressure to sedate nerve action and relieve pain in the connected organs. No use of needles has been considered necessary by him.

While various meridian lines pass through various points on the organs of the human body, all the twelve important meridians have a place in the hands and feet, as briefly indicated below :

There are three important meridians on the inner side or palm of the hand, namely : (*i*) Lung meridian, (*ii*) Pericardium meridian (also known as circulatory—sex meridian) and (*iii*) Heart meridian. There are three other important meridians on the outer side or back of the hand, namely : (*i*) Small Intestine meridian, (*ii*) Triple warmer meridian and (*iii*) Large intestine meridian.

All these six meridians have their beginnings in the finger-tips of the hands, which are important acupuncture points. On the palm side of the hand, the heart meridian starts from the tip of the small finger, the pericardium meridian from the tip of the middle finger and the lung meridian from the tip of the thumb. On the back of the hand, the small intestine meridian starts from the tip of the little finger, the triple warmer meridian from the tip of the ring finger and the large instestine meridian from the tip of the index finger.

In the case of cardiac over-work or distress, it has been recommended that pressure may be applied on the tips of the small fingers of both hands by pinching and twirling them vigorously. By doing this in an emergency, a heart attack may be alleviated and a life saved very handily.

The bottom of the foot, similarly, shows rich reflex zones and forms an integral part of the entire complex of interconnecting nerves.

There are six meridians on the foot. The bottom of the foot has three—namely : (*i*) Gall bladder meridian, (*ii*) Kidney meridian and (*iii*) Spleen meridian. There are three other meridians on the back or top of the foot—namely : (*i*) Liver meridian, (*ii*) Stomach meridian and (*iii*) Bladder meridian. The spleen meridian starts from the big toe and the kidney meridian also has its origin in the foot. All these areas play a role in enjoying good health. The toes contain the "trigger points" for head, neck as well as for ears, eyes, heart, liver, lungs and pancreas, the hollow of the foot has important points of abdomen, stomach and kidneys, while the heel accommodates important points for glands and sex organs.

It will be seen from the above that the various meridians passing through the hands and feet have connections with all the important organs of the body. Hence alleviation of pain or restoration of proper functioning of the inner organs can be easily manipulated by the application of magnets to hands and feet, as the effect of the application of magnets to the palms or soles goes to their other side also and influences all the meridians and their connected organs. Thus the correctness of the methods of application of magnets to palms and soles, suggested in Chapter 10 of this book, is verified and proved by the independent system of treatment by Acupressure.

It is interesting to note that there is a great similarity in the approach of acupressure and magnetotherapy as both the systems recommend the outwardly application on different parts of body without any internal medication. The encouraging results achieved in the treatment of various diseases through magnetotherapy, corroborate with the beneficial results obtained by acupressure. The indentical gratifying results also impart a technical verification of the clinical results of the two differen systems of treatment.

For detailed understanding of the art of acupressure and for facilitating localised application of magnets on individual acupuncture points, the readers are advised to refer to the detailed treatise on the subject of acupressure.

Suggestion for Utilising Acupuncture points in Magnetotherapy

It is suggested that the physicians who are interested in carrying out treatment by utilising acupuncture points in the body, may try the application of magnets on or near the selected points instead of pricking them with needles or applying pressure on them. It is believed that this change in their practice will give more success to them and less discomfort to their patients, as there is no piercing of needles or pressurising the points in magnetotherapy.

18

Magnetotherapy and Naturopathy

Several Branches of Naturopathy—Including Magnetotherapy

A Conference of the Indian systems of treatment including Naturopathy was held in Delhi on 25th and 26th June 1977, under the Presidentship of our Prime Minister, Shri Morarji Desai. Like Mahatma Gandhi, Shri Morarji Desai also has a great regard for and attachment with Naturopathy. The secret of his good health even after the age of 86 years lies in his natural diet, simple living and his belief in natural things.

Naturopathy includes any system of treatment with the help of natural means of recovery without drugs or surgery. It employs earth, heat, light, water, electricity, proper diet, massage and other methods. Beside, Hydropathy, Chromotherapy, Massagetherapy, Yoga and Gemtherapy are also included in Naturopathy.

State Recognition to Naturopathy

As Naturopathy is primarily an Indian system of treatment, combining several natural aids to health without drug or surgery, many State Govts. in India like Gujarat, Bihar, Tamil Nadu, Andhra Pradesh, Madhya Pradesh, Maharashtra, etc. have given this system their State recognition. And alongwith the main media of treatment, other branches included in Naturopathy are also considered to have got State recognition.

The treatment in Naturopathy through earth, heat, light, water, electricity, natural diet and massage, etc. is common and is known to almost everyone. Chromotherapy and Gemtherapy are not, however, so common. Hence information about these systems is given below :

240

Chromotherapy

Light and heat are important media of treatment in Naturopathy. Sunlight gives us both. This is an inexpensive but powerful natural agent and it plays a great part in keeping us in health, as it provides us with two important necessities of life. It is for this reason that the Sun is worshipped as God—the Protector.

Nature has provided a number of expensive methods for the preservation and also for restoration of health when it is disturbed. If it is not convenient or possible for any particular person to use mud-packs or take sun-bath, he can carry with him and take some pills having the effect of the spectral colour of Sun-rays.

Sunlight consists of several visible and invisible rays. It is safe to use visible rays for treating human diseases. The spectrum of visible rays consists of seven colours, namely : Violet, Indigo, Blue, Green, Yellow, Orange and Red. Of these, Blue, Green and Red are primary colours and the rest are mixtures thereof. The main combinations can give us over 200 hues and shades ; otherwise the seven colours can be multiplied into an unlimited number. These colours can replace hundreds of medicines in use these days.

We lose ourselves in wonder at the majesty of the perfectly ordered colours and must realize that beauty in the world is not by chance. Travlling in a plane we get only a glimpse of the cosmic vastness and the role of the Sun in the cosmic whole. The different vegetables, fruits, flowers, nuts, grains, etc,, derive their different colours from their paramount source—the Sun, which is the Supreme Power House.

It has been ascertained by the Scientists that every substance has a colour spectrum of its own. This means that every drug also has its own colour spectrum. It is, therefore, logical and has also been proved by experience that spectral colours can be used directly in place of drugs for medical effects. Thus chromotherapy uses spectral colours directly in place of conventional drugs with the result that there is no drug after-effect. Of the 7 colours mentioned above, blue is cooling and soothing, red is warming and stimulating and green is harmonising in between the two and Nature's best blood purifier.

Just as there are 3 Doshas in Ayurveda, namely : Vat, Pitta and Kaph, there are these 3 primary colours in chromotherapy. So long as the three colours are in a balanced state, a man remains in health but when this balance is upset, a state of disease is noticed.

As every medicine has some colour, every organ of the body also has some colour. For treatment in chromotherapy, the colour of the diseased organ and the temperament of the patient are ascertained and the harmonising colours are used which correct the ailments.

We have specific medicines which act directly on certain organs ; similarly there are certain colours for which different organs have affinity. Describing the affinity of every colour or every organ for a particular colour becomes a matter of detailed study which is out of the scope of this Chapter. Hence the details about the affinity are not given here.

The main medium for administration of colour effect is water but oil, sugar, candy, fruit juices and sugar milk, etc. can also be similarly charged with the colours and these things can be used for longer periods.

Method of Preparation of Solar Medicines

The healing effects of the spectral colours can be obtained by two ways :

(*i*)   by external application to the body by passing Sunlight through various coloured glass sheets, or cellophane paper, and

(*ii*) by preparing solar medicines for internal and external use.

The latter is done by exposing to sunlight, water, milk, powder, or oil, etc., stored in coloured bottles for a number of days. The medicinal effect of the colours is absorbed in the medium stored in the coloured bottles. The colour rays pass easily through water medium, so we get a medicinal charge on the water quickly—say, within eight hours of exposure to sunlight. Oils and solids have, however, to be exposed for a month or so to obtain an effective medicinal colour charge.

We have seen that, in chromotherapy, the power of the Sun is utilised through the colours of Sun-rays. In magnetotherapy, the power of magnets is made use of to cure diseases, magnets are believed to have solar power as they give heat to the body when applied to it and the magnetic waves spread out like the rays of the Sun. Hence it is evident that both the systems of treatment draw their power from the same source *i.e.* the Sun and are, therefore, alike to some extent. Moreover, just as water is charged with colours in chromotherapy, water is also charged with magnetism and magnetised water works as a good medicine in the diseases of abdomen, stomach and in urinary troubles including stones in kidneys.

Gemtherapy

Gems are the precious stones of different quality and colour and are the products of nature. The Lord of colours is the Sun. The Lord of creation is also the Sun. The Sun has bestowed life to everything on the earth through these colours and, therefore, every colour is represented by these precious stones *e.g.* Ruby, Pearl, Coral, Emerald, Topaz, Diamond and Blue-Sapphire.

In India, gems are mostly used for increasing the wealth and longivity, for power and popularity and for averting diseases and disasters. The want of anything makes one restless and perpetual restlessness consumes our energy. The loss of energy wears the garb of a disease. Gemtherapy believes, "Disease is nothing but the colour hunger". A Gemtherapist understands the colour-hunger in different diseases. If you recieve the colour which your body needs, you are cured of the disease and for this purpose you take either the radiated globules of the relevant gem or wear the gem.

There are references to gems and their power in early works on Astrology in Sanskrit. The oldest Puran, Vishnu Puran, makes elaborate observations on the origin and the power of gems. Even to this day highly ambitious people wear gems for increasing their wealth and the diseased wear them for relieving their sufferings. Gems are used all over the globe in one way or the other.

Most of the gems are used as medicine. In Ayurveda, they have been described for their use as medicine. There are elaborate processes for burning the gems and for turning them into ashes (*Bhasmas*) for administration to patients suffering from various simple and serious diseases. Undoubtedly, there is a great inherent power in gems particularly with reference to health.

The Origin of Disease

Mind controls the body and a very large percentage of diseases originates in mind. The visible expressions of the mind are emotions, namely : anger, hatred, worry, anxiety, avarice, affection, envy, fear, frustration, greed, jealousy, etc. Thse emotions put the *Chakras* (plexii) out of order and the secretions from the glands produce harmful effect and cause disease. The human being consists of body, mind and spirit and all the three need treatment—the mind is more important than the body.

The nine important gems are used for nine colours and represent nine planets as follows :

	Gem	*Colour*	*Planet*
1.	Ruby	Red	Sun
2.	Pearl	Orange, white	Moon
3.	Coral	Yellow	Mars
4.	Emerald	Green	Mercury
5.	Moon Stone (Topas)	Blue	Jupiter

6.	Diamond	Indigo	Venus
7.	Sapphire	Violet	Saturn
8.	Gomeda (Onyx)	Ultra-violet	Rahu
9.	Cat's Eye	Infra-red	Ketu

The gems always radiate cosmic colour rays. The human body is composed of cells. Every cell has its composition according to these comic rays. The state of equilibrium of these cosmic rays in the cells keeps the body healthy. When this equilibrium is disturbed, the body develops disease which can be cured by supplying deficiency of the colour ray.

How Gems Cure Diseases

Our body is composed of seven primary colours of the Solar Spectrum, namely : Violet, Indigo, Blue, Green, Yellow, Orange and Red. When there is deficiency or absence of any of these primary colours in the body, we are attacked by the diseases. For example, when red rays are absent, diseases like Anemia, Fever, Inflammation, Physical debility, Weakness, Loss of vitality, etc., invade our body. These diseases can be cured by injecting red rays into our body, by wearing or by taking the radiated globules of the gems of red planets, namely the Sun and the Mars. Their favourite gems are Ruby and Red Coral. When these gems come in contact with our body, they inject red rays into our body whereby deficiency is made up and we become free from the diseases.

Again when there is excess of red rays in our body, the excess produce diseases like boils, tumours, sun-stroke, conjunctivitis, insanity, insomnia, headache, carbuncle, etc. These diseases can be quickly cured by injecting cold rays into the body by taking globules of or by wearing cold stones. The most favourite cold stones are Moon Stone, Yellow Sapphire, White Pearl and Emerald.

Therefore, the state of equilibrium of rays is required to be maintained in our body in order to keep it healthy and free from any disease. Any excess or deficiency would result in appearance of diseases.

Each gem has abundant source of one specific rays. This source is not exhausted even after constant use of several years. That is why gems are considered most valuable healing agents. Certain gems have wonderful healing power. The most useful gems are Red Coral, White Pearl, Moon Stone, Emerald and Yellow Sapphire. Some gems are very dangerous also— for example : Ruby, Cat's Eye and Blue Sapphire, if unsuitable.

How Gems are Used in Gemtherapy

Gems are made use of in different ways in different systems of treatment. In Ayurveda, the gems are burnt into ashes and the ashes called *Bhasmas* are given to the patients with honey or with other medicines. In Unani system of tratment, the gems are ground into very thin and fine powder and are given like the *Bhasmas* of Ayurveda. Use of gems is also made in Homoeopathic way and sugar of milk globules are saturated in tinctures prepared from gems. The procedure is as follows :

An empty clean phial of 30 ml. (one ounce) is taken and one dram of rectified spirit is pured in it. The gem, medicine of which is required to be prepared, is immersed in the rectified spirit and the phial is well-corked. The phial is kept in a dark place protected from light for 7 days. The phial is then taken out and given good shakes. The rectified spirit is transferred to another phial of 30 ml. and homoeopathic blank globules are added to the spirit. By gentle rotation of the phial all the globules are saturated with the gem remedy. The medicine of the particular gem is then ready for use. The gem may be preserved safely for being utilised similarly later on. The gem does not lose its power or effect and may be used as many times as required.

If medicine of more than one gem is required to be prepared, all the gems concerned may be immersed in the rectified spirit together and the same procedure may be followed.

Magnetotherapy helps in Meditation

Naturopathy brings about a balance of the mind adding to the power of concentration. The same can be achieved through

Magnetotherapy also. Experiments have shown that the use of magnets helps in meditation by creating an equilibrium in the mental nerves. In this regard, the following facts are mentionable :

(1) Magnetic energy provides substance and strength to the net-work of nervous system thereby giving initiative and depth to the power of concentration and meditation. Application of magnets has helped in Transcendental Meditation also.

(2) Magnetism regulates the process of blood circulation and energises the digestive system. It provides the body with necessary heat. Thus magnetism preserves complete health of the *Sadhak* and provides him with requisite physical and mental environment for meditation.

(3) Magnetism dispenses the accumulation in the body of foreign elements like Calcium, Cholesterol, etc., and thus releases the tension in nerves. It renders the body flexible—an essential condition for practising Yoga.

(4) Magnetism gives strength and normalcy to the functions of mind, heart and lungs and has direct effect on respiratory system. Thus it heips in *Pranayam* and Yogic practices relating to breathing.

(5) Magnetism is very helpful in purging human physical mechanism of all unwanted elements through excertions thereby giving to whole system a balanced activity devoid of excitement.

It will be observed from the above that Magnetism is prone to exercise a deep effect on all inner and outer workings of the body. Magnetotherapy can thus prove a valuable aid to the family men and Yogis alike.

As Magnetism releases strain and tension in nerves and provides them with requisite energy, therefore, intellectuals like Judges, Advocates. Vakils, Professors, Writers, Secretaries, Business Executives and Mental Workers also are sure to be benefitted by the regular use of magnets. Even 5 minutes magnet-touch in the morning means a natural exercise and will keep them physically fit, active and energetic as well as mentally alert. Hence everyone should take this exercise in his/her home regularly. It is beneficial for these who cannot get out for morning walks or do any other exercise. It works as a preventive too against many ailments which may otherwise come.

Ponts of Similarity between Magnetotherapy and Naturopathy

Magnetotherapy, in its spirit and content, is quite similar to Naturopathy, so much so that the former could be considered a branch of the latter. Naturopathy, as practised today, can be substantially supplemented through the application of magnetism. Just as the earth, water and electricity are the agents of healing in Naturopathy, magnetic energy which is the medium in Magnetotherapy is as good as direct gift and force of Nature as electricity is. To stress these points further, several points of similarties between these two systems are given below :

(1) Magnetotherapy is a system of treatment of various diseases through application of magnets to the body of the patients just as Naturopathy is a system of treatment with application of earth, electricity, heat, light, water, etc.

(2) Magnetotherapy is an external treatment and is carried out by applying magnets to the body externally, just a naturopathy is an external treatment carried out by applying heat, light, water, massage, etc., externally.

(3) No drugs or surgery are administered in magnetotherapy just as no drugs or surgery are given in Naturopathy. Both are drugless systems of treatment.

(4) Magnetotherapy regulates blood-circulation, autonomic nervous system as well as other systems working in the body, namely : digestive, respiratory, urinogenital, just as naturopathy improves and regulates all these systems.

(5) Magnetic treatment produces heat in the body and goes a long way to relieve pains, swelling, stiffness, etc., besides many other diseases like eczema and spondylitis. Electric treatment also works in the same way and both the treatments are, therefore, similar.

(6) There are no adverse effects in the treatment of magnetotherapy as there are no ill after-effects in Naturopathy.

(7) No big machinery or apparatuses are required in the treatment of Magnetotherapy ; only a few pairs of magnets are sufficient to treat all diseases. Naturopathy also does not need big machinery and apparatuses and they are accordingly similar.

(8) Magnetotherapy is quite simple, safe and economical like Naturopathy. There is no recurring expenditure in magnetotherapy as the same magnets can be used for hundreds of patients for various diseases and for years together. If the magnets lose some of their strength in the course of time (4-5 years), they can be recharged to regain their lost strength and become active again.

(9) Magnetotherapy pleads for the use of magnetised water in almost all diseases—especially all stomach and urinary trobles—just as water is made use of, to a great extent, in Naturopathy.

(10) Electricity and magnetism are two branches of a natural force. Electricity is already included in Naturopathy. Magnetism also plays a great part in curing diseases of almost all kinds and should, therefore, be considered to be a medium of treatment in Naturopathy.

Some Preferential Points in Magnetotherapy

1. The time required for magnet-treatment, everyday as well as on the whole, is much less than the time required for treatment by every branch of Naturopathy, every day as well as for the whole treatment.

2. The magnet-treatment is much cheaper than the treatment of Naturopathy in its different branches.

3. There are no or very limited precautions or restrictions in Magnetotherapy in the matter of diet, eating and drinking habits and other movements, etc., while Naturopathy puts in many restrictions in these respects.

4. The magnet-treatment can be easily taken at one's residence if the patient has the required magnets with him, while it is not easily possible to take Naturopathy treatment at home in many cases—particularly with electric machines.

Conclusion

The position explained above evidently shows that Magnetotherapy is a natural treatment and even has some preferential points over Naturopathy. But it is not considered to be a part of Naturopathy so far. It would be in the fitness of things now if Magnetotherapy is recognised by all Naturopaths, Naturopathy Associations and the State and Central Governments, as a branch of Naturopathy. The recognition will benefit both Naturopathy as well as Magnetotherapy. Naturopathy will be enriched further by magnet-treatment and Magnetotherapy will have more support of public as well as recognition by Governments.

19

Electromagnetotherapy

We have so far dealt with the use of permanent magnets in magnetotherapy as they have remained the chief tools of treatment in the hands of the magnetotherapists for quite a long time.

The usefulness of electromagnets has remained restricted to the technical, mechanical and industrial spheres in the past but their therapeutic capabilities and several advantages over the permanent magnets have recently been realised and are now being utilised for the purpose of curing different diseases.

Limitations of Magnetotherapy

During the course of application of permanent magnets, the magnetotherapists found some limitations in this system of treatment, namely :

(1) The strength of the magnets and the speed of their working is always static and cannot be decreased or increased according to the requirement of the case.

(2) The recovery from and the cure of the disease takes long time, while the patient of today is quite impatient and wants immediate relief, irrespective of the length of his disease.

(3) Experience shows that patients come to test magnetotherapy, as a last resort, when they have tried almost all the known systems of treatment, namely : Allopathy, Homoeopathy, Ayurvedic and Unani systems and have not been benefitted by them. Nevertheless, they expect that this new and specialised system should give them immediate relief to some extent at least.

251

Giving due consideration to all these factors, magnetotherapists have adopted Electromagnets in their practice.

Electromagnet too has some of its own limitations, for example it cannot work without electricity, it should not be applied on very tender organs of body like eyes. Hence an electromagnet cannot be a complete substitute for permanent magnet and therefore both of them have to exist simultaneously, so that either of them may be utilised according to its suitability for every case.

It has been noticed that the effect of an electromagnet on the human body is more penetrating, fast healing and long-lasting, especially in the cases of chronic diseases *e.g.* arthritis, backache, fractures, gout, lumbago, paralysis, poliomyelitis, sciatica, spondylitis, slipped disc, etc. Hence the attention of the magnetotherapists was drawn to it, and a large number of them has adopted it.

The difference between the two kinds of magnets is only technical and both these types are to exist as complementary to each other as therapeutic magnetic tools.

What is an Electromagnet

When a bar or any other piece of soft iron is placed inside a solenoid (cylindrical coil of insulated wire) carrying an electric current, it gets magnetised and behaves as a magnet as long as the current is on. When the current is switched off, the magnetism disappears and the piece of iron reverts to its original unmagnetised state, while magnetism in a permanent magnet is a static phenomenon. The strength of electromagnet can either be increased or decreased with the help of a regulator. This is a definite advantage of electromagnet over permanent magnet.

Electromagnets of Various Strengths

Electromagnets can be made in various sizes, designs and strength. Big and high powered electromagnets are usually harnessed for industry, but only small electromagnets of less strength are used for medical and other purposes. They can be of any shape and size *viz.* : oval, square, rectangular or cylindrical. The standard electromagnets used for the purpose of treatment are fitted with regulators for effecting increase or decrease in their strength according to the requirements of the case.

An indicator lamp is provided on such electromagnets which is automatically switched on when the current starts flowing in the device and is switched off when the current is discontinued. Small round electromagnets are made for medical purposes and they have only one or two strength. They are sufficient for treatment of general ailments.

A.C. or D.C. Electromagnets

Electromagnets can be made with and can work on Alternating Current (AC) as well as with Direct Current (DC). It is considered that the magnets made with alternating current work better and give more beneficial and quicker results. The reason is that ripples or pulsations are formed in the working of AC magnets and with the change of poles, the cells and tissues are stirred vigorously and they produce better healing effect as compared with the static effect of permanent magnets. AC electromagnets are thus more useful for treatment of chronic diseases like arthritis, pains, swellings and bone diseases and more practitioners are, therefore, using AC electromagnets.

An electromagnet used with alternating current, when applied to the diseased part of the body, given 50 strokes or knocks of the North pole and an equal number of strokes of South pole alternately in one second, which means 3000 strokes in one minute. The strokes are so quick that the patient is unable to feel any difference between the strokes, he feels only pulsations.

The electromagnetic strokes penetrate deep into bones, bone-marrow and muscles and give appreciable relief and soothing effect to muscles and nerves.

Electric Shock Therapy

The electromagnetic treatment is quite different in effect

and nature from the electric shock-therapy. The electric shocks **are** shocking but not soothing, they are intense but do not go deeper than the surface and they can be injurious if prolonged even by a second. In contrast to this, the electromagnetic strokes are all along positive, healing and soothing. They give intense relief to the nerves, and are quite harmless in effect.

Application of Electromagnets

Electromagnets are not used alone but they are applied in conjuction with premier magnets. The premier magnets **are** applied in accordance with the nature and place of the disease. They are applied to the affected parts of the body or to the hands or feet of the patients on the lines of the treatment with permanent magnets. Important places in the body, where electromagnets are applied for treatment of various diseases, **are** almost the same as suggested in the books on magnetotherapy.

Electromagnets are utilised in treatment of chronic diseases as well as in acute ailments and they give good results even in cases given up by other systems of treatment. Some magneto-therapists have also selected neck, epigastrium and centre of back where premier and electromagnets may be applied in addition to the palms of hands and the soles of feet.

However, the magnetotherapists should make use of their own experience and skill and consider the nature and place of the disease and the pole of the magnets before giving the electro-magnetic treatment.

Use of Specific Permanent Magnets with Eletromagnets

At our centre the use of an electromagnet is combined with the use of specific permanent magnets in order to get the full effect of the treatment. The polarity of the permanent magnet to be used with the electromagnet should be determined accord-ing to the principles of treatment with permanent magnets.

In our experience, the round and flat magnets, encased in thick and scratch-resistant ABS (High Quality Plastic), introduced by our centre and called premier magnets, are proving very

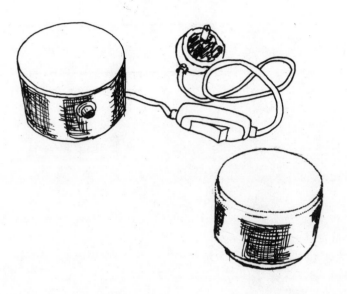

Electromagnet with Premier Magnet

useful for this electromagnetic treatment. A premier magnet has both the poles on opposite sides and any pole of it can be used according to the nature of the disease. The selected pole of the premier magnet is applied to the diseased part of the body and the electromagnet is placed quite near the premier magnet or in between two premier magnets or on opposite side of the place of disease.

Mental Satisfaction

By applying permanent magnets, the patient does not feel any sensation or effect of the magnet but when an electromagnet is applied or is placed near a premier or ceramic magnet or between two such magnets, the patient immediately feels the magnetic pulsations and experiences the effect of eletromagnetism in his body, creating a soothing and direct influence on his system. Besides the greater physical benefits, this treatment gives mental satisfaction also as the patient readily feels that electromagnetic activity is going on in his body where the magnets have been applied.

Duration of Electromagnetic Treatment

The time for treatment is usually from 5 minutes to 10 minutes, depending upon the strength of the patient and the power of the electromagnet used for the treatment. The treatment should be started with lesser duration, which may be increased gradually up to the maximum period mentioned above.

Precautions during Electromagnetic Treatment

All precautions advised in respect of treatment with permanent magnets should be observed during electromagnetic treatment also.

Some Cases Treated by the Author

1. A 50 years old high official of the Government of India had suffered from cervical spondylosis for about 22 years and had taken almost all types of treatments (allopathic, homoeopathic, Ayurvedic, etc.), but could not get permanent relief. One of his friends suggested magnetotherapy to him and he consulted me. I assured him of relief and cure provided he took the treatment regularly for a considerable period.

He used to feel pain in cervical vertebrae 3, 4 and 5, which extended to both of his shoulders. To begin with, high power magnets were applied on the affected area for about 10 days which did not have any effect on him. Then I switched over to electromagnet and premier magnets. I applied the electromagnet to the affected vertebrae alongwith two premier magnets—One on each of his shoulders. North pole on the back of right shoulder and South pole on the back of left shoulder for 15 minutes everyday. He took this treatment for about one month regularly and started feeling better. Unfortunately, due to his tour to Europe and USA he could not take the treatment any longer. I could not expect this result with permanent magnets alone, in such a chronic case.

2. A 35-36 years old lady suffering from frozen shoulder of left side, for the past one year, visited my clinic. She was not able to raise her left arm. She had taken all sorts of treatment including massages with medicated oils but with no effect. She was advised by one of her relatives to give a trial to magnetotherapy for some time. She agreed and used to visit my clinic for magnetic treatment from a distance of about twenty kilometres everyday.

One premier magnet (North pole) was applied to the upper part of her left arm and another premier magnet (South pole) on the lower side of her left arm at a distance of about 5-6 inches. The electro-magnet was placed in between the two premier magnets. She used to feel strong vibrations at both the places where premier magnets were applied. She took this treatment regularly for about three weeks. After each sitting she used to feel better and further better. After a fortnight, she could raise her hand to a considerable height, without much difficulty.

3. Smt. A of New Delhi working in the Ministry of Health, aged 48 years, had been suffering from acute pain in her right knee for the past 3 years and had a lot of difficulty in movements due to this pain although she was never bed-ridden. She applied electromagnet alongwith one premier magnet on the right knee for about 10 minutes daily. In about 10-12 days she found a lot of relief and in about one and a half month's

time, she was almost cured. However, on my advice she continued the treatment for some time more.

4. Smt. B of New Delhi, aged 47 years, suffered from severe backache and pain in her knees. She had already tried the modern medicine alongwith some ayurvedic medicine but pain persisted. She took magnetic treatment. One electromagnet and two premier magnets were applied to her back for ten minutes, with the help of her son who used to hold them at the proper places. North pole of one premier magnet was applied on the right side of her back and South pole of another premier magnet on the left side of her back where she felt the pain. The eletromagnet was placed between the two premier magnets, This treatment was given for about 10 minutes almost every day.

For the treatment of her knee pain, South pole of the Premier magnets was placed on the point of pain and electro-magnet about one centimeter away, for about 5-6 minutes, on each knee. She was completely relieved of her backache as well as of her knee pain in about a month.

5. Shri X of New Delhi, aged 65 years had fractured the last finger of his right hand in an accident in January 1984. He came to this clinic fifteen days after the removal of the plaster. He had swelling and pain on both sides of the right hand (on dorsal as well as the palm side). He was given electromagnetic treatment for 5 minutes near the finger which improved considerably in a week's time.

6. Shri Y of New Delhi, aged 72 years got an attack of paralysis on the right side (Hemiplegia). Both of his right arm and right leg were affected. He was taking treatment elsewhere but with no effect. One of his friends suggested to go in for magnetotherapy.

He was neither in a position to come to my clinic nor to purchase the high power magnets. He could arrange only one piece of premier magnets which he applied regularly. He was advised to keep his right palm on the North pole and right sole on the South pole of the magnet for about half an hour every-day. As a result of this treatment for about two months, weak-ness of the limbs reduced considerably, and he felt sure that he would be alright by this treatment, without the use of electro magnet.

METHOD OF TREATMENT

Some common diseases and the places at which Premier and Electro-magnets are applied together, with the pole of the premier magnet, are noted below for information :

1. Arthritis : North pole of premier magnet on the affected place and electromagnet near the premier magnet.

2. Asthma : A special treatment has been given at the end of this list.

3. Backache : South pole of P.M. on spot of pain or on lumbar region & electromagnet by its side.

4. Bronchitis, influenza : As for Asthma.

5. Constipation : N.P. of P.M. on navel & S.P. on lumbar region. Electro M. on both the places separately. near P.M.

6. Diabetes : N.P. of P.M. on Pancreas and S.P. of P.M. on back (opposite to N.P.) Electro M. near both the poles separately.

7. Diarrhea/Dysentery : N.P. of P.M. on navel & S.P. on lumbar region with Electro M. near each pole separately.

8. Fracture : N.P. of P.M. on the affected bone & electro M. by its side. If the fracture extends to some inches in length, N.P. on the upper part and the S.P. on the lower part with Electro M. between both the poles.

9. Headache : N.P. of ceramic magnet on right temple and S.P. of ceramic magnet on left temple with Electro M. on cheek of each side for 5 minutes only.

10. Hernia : S.P. of P.M. on Hernia and Electro M. by its side.

11. Hypertension (H.B.P.) : N.P. of P.M. touching the right pulse; Electro M. on the other side of wrist.

12. Hypotension (L.B.P.) : S.P. of P.M. touching left pulse & Electro M. on the other side of wrist.

13. Haemorrhoids (Piles) : N.P. of P.M. on spot or sacral region and Electro M. by its side.

14. Kidney troubles (including stone) : S.P. of P.M. on renal region & Electro M. by its side.

15. Nervousness : S.P. of P.M. on back of neck & Electro M. near it.

16. Neuralgia : S.P. of P.M. on painful spot & Electro M. near or on opposite side.

17. Obesity : N.P. of P.M. near navel & S.P. on middle of back & Electro M. with each P.M. separately.

18. Palpitation (Cardiac anxiety and weakness) : N.P. of P.M. near the heart, S.P. of P.M. on back side of heart region & Electro M. near each pole separately for five minutes only.

19. Paralysis : Right palm of patient on N.P. of P.M. & Electro M. on dorsal side (back) of palm of affected side & S.P. of P.M. under sole with Electro M. on dorsal side of foot of affected foot. If arms and legs of both the sides are affected, the same treatment should be given to both sides separately.

20. Prostate gland : S.P. of P.M. on bladder or gland & Electro M. near the P.M.

21. Rheumatism : S.P. of P.M. on painful part & Electro M. near it. If pain extends to several parts, the same treatment should be given to each part separately.

22. Sciatica : N.P. of P.M. on upper part of affected leg from where pain starts, with Electro M. near it, and S.P. of P.M. under sole with electro M. on upper side of foot.

23. Polio : N.P. of P.M. on affected hip and S.P. of P.M. under affected sole with Electro M. near each magnet separately.

24. Stiff Shoulders : N.P. of P.M. on front side on affected shoulder and Electro M. near it and S.P. of the P.M. on back of shoulder with Electro M. near it .

25. Tumors : N.P. of P.M. on the tumor & Eleclro M. near it.

Magnetised water is a great help and necessary supplement to the main treatment by the application of magnets. Drinking water should, therefore, be magnetised with the H.P.M., M.P.M. or P.M., whichever magnets are available. It should be given 3-4 times every day in the quantity of 2 to 3 ounces at a time.

An Expert Opinion about Electromagnetic Treatment

Dr. A.K. Rakshit, consulting physician of magneto-medicine, London, has made the following statement :

"The Medical Electro-Biology is a non-invasive form of treatment, successfully used in Degenerative Osteo-Arthrosis, non-union of bones, fractures and sports injuries. It has also many other applications in place of internal medicine, psychiatry as well as oncology".

ASTHMA AND BRONCHITIS TREATMENT
TWO METHODS

I.   (i) N.P. of P.M. under right palm, & Electro M. on back of right palm.

(ii) S.P. of P.M. under left palm & Electro M. on back of left palm.

5 minutes each, one by one.

II.   (i) N P. of P.M. on Back of right side of chest.

(ii) S.P. of P.M. on back of left side of chest.

(iii) Electro M. on back, between both the P.Ms.

Simultaneously for 10 minutes.

Both the treatments can be given to a patient. Treatment No. I in the morning and treatment No. II in the evening or at night while lying in bed.

Part VIII

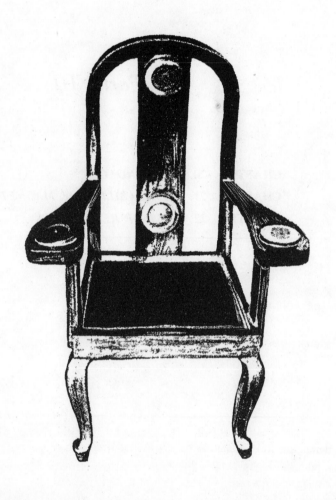

MAGNETIC CHAIR: fitted with four strong magnets, used for Cervical Spondylitis, slipped disc, backache, etc...

20

Terminology

Technical Terms relating to Magnet and Magnetism

Several technical terms relating to magnetism have been used in this book. An explanation of such terms will help the reader in the proper understanding of the subject matter. Some of the terms have already been explained in the text. The meanings of some others are given below :

Animal Magnetism

Hypnotism or mesmerism.

Biomagnetics

The science of processes and functions in living organism induced by the static magnetic fields.

Coercive Force

The capacity or power of a magnetised material to resist demagnetising influences. It is more difficult to demagnetise a material having high coercive power than to demagnetise that having low coercive power.

Electromagnetism

A branch of science which treats of the relation of electricity to magnetism. Also, magnetic action induced by an electric current.

Gauss

The unit of magnetic flux density. (After the name of J.K.F. Gauss). (Please see the note at the end of this chapter).

Hypnotism

The art or science of inducing a sleep-like state in which the mind responds to the external suggestion of the 'Agent' and can recover forgotten memories.

Keepers

Soft iron pieces connected with the different poles of magnets so that the latter do not lose their magnetism. The soft iron pieces become induced magnets closing the molecular chain so that there are no free poles to get demagnetised in course of time.

Magnet

A body or piece of iron, steel or alloy, to which the properties of attraction and repulsion have been imparted and which possesses the quality of attracting iron particles to itself.

Magnet, Ceramic

A magnet made of any synthetic material like the potter's clay, iron-oxide, etc., or any other product that is first shaped and then hardened by means of heat and then magnetised.

Magnet, Metallic (Cast-alloy)

A magnet made of any metal such as iron, steel, etc. or of a mixture of metals called cast-alloy.

Magnetic Field

The space surrounding a magnet over which magnetic force it felt. The space is permeated by magnetic lines of force. The magnetic field is most intense near the poles of the magnet.

Magnetic Flush

A sudden, swift and vigorous flow of magnetic power.

Magnetic Flux

The discharge or flow of magnetic force or the magnetic field intensity.

Magnetic Induction

Magnetisation of a magnetic material when placed in proximity with a magnetic force, without actual contact with the magnet.

Magnetic Lines of Force

Continuous curve-lines in the magnetic field showing the direction of the magnetic force and the value of intensity for every point surrounding a magnet. Externally, the lines join North pole to South pole and internally they pass from South pole to North pole. The lines of force never intersect at any point.

Magnetic Material

Substances or materials such as iron, steel, nickel, cobalt or any alloy, which are appreciably attracted by a magnet and can retain magnetism.

Magnetic Permeability

When a magnetic material is magnetised by induction, the lines of force of the magnetising field get concentrated inside the material. The degree to which the lines of force can penetrate or permeate the material is known as its permeability. In other words, the ratio of flux density to magnetising force.

Magnetisation

The act of rendering anything magnetic or imparting the property of attraction and repulsion to anything.

Magnetised Water

Water permeated with magnetic force by continuous contact with a magnet.

Magnetism

The science which deals with the properties of magnet, namely, attraction and repulsion. The power of a magnet to attract or repel other magnetic material.

Magnometer

The apparatus used for measuring Magnetic field intensities.

Magnetotherapy

The science and art of treatment of various diseases through the medium of magnets.

Mesmerism

Animal magnetism. Hypnotism, as expounded by Mesmer—a German physician.   Hypnotic suggestions or influence.

Oersted

The unit of magnetic field strength.   (Named in honour of Hans Christian Oersted).   (Please see the note at the end of this chapter).

Personal Magnetism

Power of a personality to make itself felt and to exercise its influence on others.

Polarisation

The act of acquiring or giving polarity, or developing new meanings and qualities.

Pole

The extremity of any axis about which forces acting on it are symmetrically disposed. One of the two points in a magnet, cell or battery having opposite physical qualities.

North Pole

The end of the earth's axis in the Arctic region.   The direction in which the North pole of a pivoted magnet will point.

South Pole

The end of the earth's axis in Antarctica.   The direction in which the South pole of a pivoted magnet will point.

Psychiatry

That branch of medicine which treats of mental and neurotic diseases and the pathologic or psychopathological changes associated with them.

Psychoanalysis

A method of investigation and psychotherapy whereby nervous diseases or mental ailments are traced to be forgotten, hidden concepts in the patient's mind and treated by bringing them to light.

Note : The unit of magnetic intensity was formerly known as the "GAUSS", which term is still used by some manufacturers and users of magnets. The unit is, however, called the "Oersted" now, according to the recommendations of the International Conference on Physics held in London in 1934. Some persons use the abbreviation "Oe" for the term "Oersted". ☐☐☐

ABBREVIATIONS USED IN THIS BOOK STAND FOR

N.P.	—	North pole
S.P.	—	South pole
P.M.	—	Premier magnets
H.P.	—	High power
M.P.	—	Medium power
M.W.	—	Magnetised water
Electro M.	—	Electromagnet

21

Availability of Magnets

The author, through his long experience and practice in the employment of industrial, educational and other magnets in various types, shapes and strength for the treatment of varied ailments, has selected three types of magnets. Special care has been taken to measure the gauss power of these magnets for their suitability for different age-groups, organs of the body and ailments. The use of these three types of magnets has been standardised depending upon the age of the patient and the length and severity of the disease.

With a view to make these magnets long-lasting, more effective and easy to handle, the cast-alloy magnets are encased in steel covers. The encasement increases the power of magnets several times. They are also so designed as to be compact, sturdy and befitting for local and general treatment. These magnets are, consequently, quite suitable for the entire range of ailments and patients.

The author, therefore, uses these encased cast-alloy magnets. These are generally used in pairs and in two different strengths, namely, (*i*) about 1500 gauss and (*ii*) about 2800—3000 gauss. He also uses ceramic magnets of lesser strength in curved shape (crescent type) in pairs without encasement.

The following magnets are used by the author and can be supplied by this Centre :

No. 1. Ceramic Magnets (Crescent Type) Ordinary/Delux

Ordinary magnets in black colour, Deluxe magnets in two colours :

North pole BLUE and South pole ORANGE.

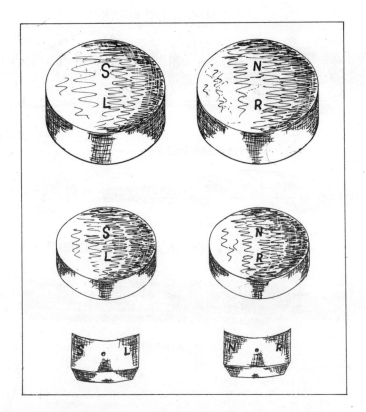

(Top Row) High Power Cast Alloy Magnets
Iron weight-lifting capacity — 10 kg, used for diseases of Adults.

(Middle Row) Medium Power Cast Alloy Magnets
Iron weight-lifting capacity — 5 kg., used for boys and girls between 3 and 16 years.

(Bottom Row) Low Power Crescent type Ceramic Magnets
used for curved organs, such as eyes, ears, nose, throat, etc., and for children upto 3 years.

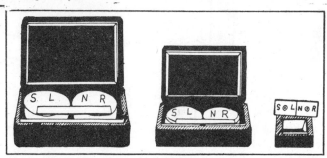

These three type of pairs of Magnets are supplied in beautiful wooden boxes.

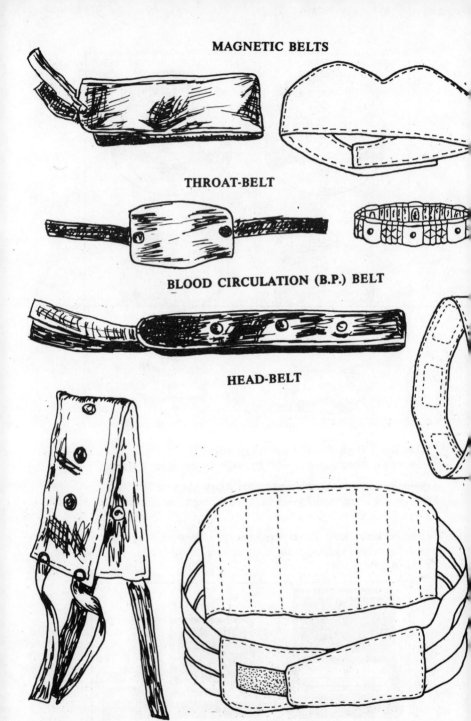

MAGNETIC BELTS

THROAT-BELT

BLOOD CIRCULATION (B.P.) BELT

HEAD-BELT

KNEE-BELT

STOMACH OR BELLY BELT

Suitable for application to curved places in the body, namely, chin, ears, eyes, nose, teeth, throat and for small children upto the age of 3 years.

No. 2. Cast Alloy, Medium Power Magnets

Suitable for local and general application in the case of elder children upto the age of 14-15 years and for other weak persons.

Round and flat—Encased in steel covers.

Strength about 1500 gauss.

No. 3. Cast Alloy, High Power or Strong Magnets

Suitable for local and general application in the case of diseases of adults.

Round and flat—Encased in steel covers.

Strength about 2800-3000 gauss.

All these three types of magnets are supplied in pairs. These magnets and different kinds of magnetic belts and necklaces for the treatment of ailments of various parts of body, kept in beautiful wooden boxes are available from :

All the products shown in the book have been redesigned by us and several new ones have been added . For full details please contact:

Pjan International, Inc.

P.O. BOX 1697,

Redondo Beach, CA 90278.

1-800-438-7736.

22

List of References

1. *Todays Health Guide*
   Published by the American Medical Association.

2. *Physiological Basis of Medical Practice*
   by C.H. Best and N.B. Taylor, Sixth Edition (1955)
   The Williams & Wilkins Company, Baltimore.

3. *Clinical Unipolar Electrocardiography*
   by B.S. Lipman and Edward, Massie, Third Edition,
   The Year Book Publishers Inc. Chicago, U.S.A.

4. *The Story of Psychoanalysis*
   by Lucy Freeman and Marvin Small, cardinal edition.
   Pocket Books, Inc. New York.

5. *Human Anatomy and Physiology*
   by V. Tatarinov, MIR Publications, Moscow (1971).

6. *Biological Effects of Magnetic Fields*
   Edited by Madeleine F. Barnothy, Professor of Physics,
   University of Illinois, U.S.A. Volumes I & II,
   Plenum Press, New York (1974 Edition).

7. *Organon of Medicine, Sixth Edition*
   by Dr. Samuel Hahnemann, Founder of Homoeopathy,
   B. Jain Publishers (P) Ltd., New Delhi-110055

8. *Materia Medica Pura, Volume II*
   by Dr. S. Hahnemann. Published by B. Jain Publishers
   (P) Ltd., New Delhi-110055.

9. *Materia Medica of Nosodes* (*with Proving of the X-Ray*)
   by Dr. H.C. Allen, M.D. Published by B. Jain Publishers
   (P) Ltd., New Delhi-110055.

10. *Key Notes and Characteristics with Comparisons of some of the Leading Remedies*
    by Dr H.C. Allen. Published by B. Jain Publishers (P) Ltd., New Delhi-110055.

11. *Magnet and Magnetic Fields or Healings by Magnets*
    by Dr A.R. Davis of America and Dr A.K. Bhattacharya of Naihati, West Bengal. Published by Firma K.L. Mukhopadhyay, Banchharam Akrur Lane, Calcutta.

12. *Secrets of Magnet Therapy—The Acknowledged Science of Natural Healing and Cure*
    by Dr H.T. Bolakani of Bombay (Not a priced publication).

13. *Abstract of Bio-magnetics Symposium in Japan*
    Published by Aimante Mfg. Co. Ltd., Tokyo, Japan.

14. *Clinical Effects of Magnetic Health Bands on the so-called "Stiff shoulders"*
    by Tabata National Railway Hospital, Japan.

15. *Magazine "Life", International,* April 1963.

16. *Magazines "Soviet Land",* No. 20 of October 1970 and *"Soviet Union"* No. 8 of 1973.

17. *Magazine "Participant Journal",* January 1972.

18. *Magazine "Bhavan's Journal",* Volume XIX, No. 17, dated 18-3-73. Published from Bombay.

19. *About Yoga—The Complete Philosophy*
    by Harvey Day (1956) Published by Thorsons Publishers Ltd. St. Martins Lane, London.

20. *Sant Darshan, Yogic Chamatkar Chapter*
    Published by Vishwa Gyan Mandir, Kankhal (Distt. Saharanpur, U.P.).

21. *Holy Bible—New Testament—Gospel according to the St. Methew—*Chapters 8 and 9. The Gideons International, Chicago II, Illinois, U.S.A.

22. *Acupuncture*
    by Dr Felix Mann, *MB of England, Vintage Books Edition 1973,* Random House, New York.

23. *Acupressure*
    by Dr J.V. Cerney of U.S.A. (1975 reprint), Cornerstone
    Library Publications, New York.

24. *The Science of Medicine and Physiological Concepts in Recent
    and Medieval India*, edited by Dr N.H. Keswani, Dean,
    Professor and Head of Department of Anatomy and History
    of Medicine, All India Institute of Medical Sciences, New
    Delhi (1974). Published by the National Book Trust,
    Government of India.

25. *Three Thousand Years of Magnets*
    by V.P. Kartsev, *English Translation* by MIR Publishers,
    Moscow (1975)

26. *The Times of India and the Hindustan Times*, Daily News-
    papers of New Delhi.

27. *Science Reporter* for June, 1977
    Magnetic Fields in Human Body
    Council of Scientific and Industrial Research,
    New Delhi.

28. IEEE Transactions on Magnets, Vol. MAG-11, No. 6.
    Nov. 1975. High Gradient Magnetic Separation of Red
    Cells from whole blood and No. 135/1975/Spectrum/5 by
    Dr D. Melville, Southampton University.

29. *Eve's Weekly*, January 7-13, 1978

30. *Soviet Land*, No. 8 for April, 1978

31. *Magnet-Therapy*, by Dr Neville S. Bengali of Bombay,
    B. Jain Publishers (P) Ltd., New Delhi-110055.

□ □ □

Index

273